Who Stole My Food? ©

Over a Trillion dollars per year for Chronic Diseases...

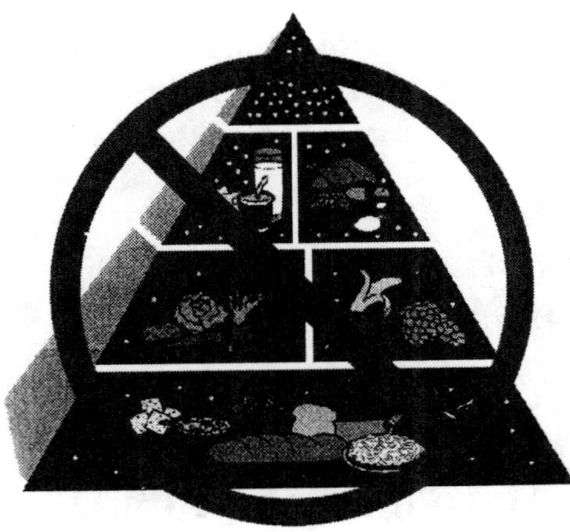

...caused by the bad recommendations in the Food Pyramids *and* Food Guidelines

Harold Rongey, Ph.D.

Who Stole My Food? is intended solely to inform and educate on matters concerning nutrition as it relates to health. and bodily functions, and not as personal medical advice. Please consult your doctor or medical professional if you have questions regarding your medical condition. If your questions are in regards to nutrition as it relates to your health, it may be a good idea to determine the level of his or her training in the field of nutrition — some medical schools no longer teach courses in nutrition. Some schools do offer such courses as electives to pre-medical students.

Who Stole My Food?

Cover, Book Design, and Illustrations by:
Cheryl Hayes-Burger

Library of Congress Cataloging-in-Publication Data
ISBN

Harold Rongey, Ph.D.

Published by R/B Publishing, LLC
Placentia, CA

For information regarding special discounts for bulk purchases, please see back of book.

Who Stole My Food? ©

For your information, I declare that:

I am not affiliated with any organizations, research. facilities, or companies involved in any way with the medical professions or health. services. I am an independent scientist, concerned with having the world become healthier through better nutrition. The philosophy expressed in this book represents my own theories pertaining to the cause of chronic diseases, and how they might be prevented or cured. Should you choose to follow any part of my philosophy, you are advised to consult your medical professional(s) before doing so.

However, if your professional is good at “soft shoe” dancing around the questions, you may benefit by finding a more knowledgeable professional to guide you.

To

Humanity

"Life is not merely to be alive, but to be well". ~Marcus Valerius Martial

Table of Contents

Acknowledgement

This book is a salute to those dedicated scientists and physicians who, for the first half of the 20th century, determined the nutritional needs for man and other species of animals. They were diligent, basing their research. on sound scientific studies using the Scientific Method. You may gain a better understanding of the Scientific Method by reading one of the many books written on this subject or reading the description of the Scientific Method presented by Dr. Ravnskov, M.D., Ph.D. in The Cholesterol. Myths.(38)

Until the late 1950s the research standards of testing were quite laborious. It was often found that the hypotheses being tested had to be revised multiple times to confirm that the factor under study was indeed the cause of disease, and capable of disease prevention or possibly cure. This included vitamins such as vitamin C in the prevention of scurvy, or folic acid in the prevention of neural tube defect or spina bifida plus many others as they relate to other diseases.

They identified the vitamins, minerals, amino acids, proteins, carbohydrates, fatty acids, and fiber essential for good nutrition. They isolated them, and determined the specific needs for each species. This gave rise to the Recommended Daily Allowance (RDAs) by the National Institutes of Health, National Academy of Sciences/National Research Council (NIH/NAS/NRC) for each species, including humans.

The United States Department of Agriculture (USDA) began compiling data on the composition of foods in the early 1900s. Today you will find this data base represents one of the better data sources, and includes not only the basic foods, but most all of the manufactured foods available for human or animal consumption. The work of those individuals is truly commendable when one considers the analytical tools available during the first half of the 20th century. The second half of the 20th century has confirmed the value of their efforts. The healthy and profitable farm animals have had their diets formulated to the RDAs since the late 1940s. Domestic pets and exotic animals have healthier, longer lives as well, due to diets formulated to the RDAs since 1973. In the mid 1940s through the late 1950s they were showing much success with humans, using RDA based vitamin and mineral supplements combined with good foods. (This approach for humans was abandoned in the late 1950s.)

Special Thanks

I owe a great debt of gratitude to those who have assisted in the preparation of this book through their many suggestions and recommendations which have made the book more understandable. They are:
my wife Verna, Cheryl Hayes-Burger, and Sheila Norris.

Authors Forward

The overall picture to be considered here is the tremendous annual cost for the total medical services performed in this country. The rates at which these costs are expanding, in comparison to the growing numbers of individuals having to live with non-infectious, chronic diseases, is shocking and out of control. The Centers for Disease Control and Prevention (CDC).reported that in year 2000 our total medical costs in the U.S. were over one trillion dollars per year, and seventy-five percent (75%) of this cost is related to chronic diseases.

More recently, in 2006 the total medical costs were reported to be two trillion dollars, with no end in sight for the continued increasing costs. (26) There are over a thousand such diseases including arthritis, attention deficit disorder, attention deficit hyperactivity disorder, lupus, Parkinson's, numerous cancers, multiple sclerosis, muscular dystrophy, coronary heart disease, aneurisms, gout, type II diabetes, hypertension, strokes, arteriosclerosis, schizophrenia, bipolar disorder, etc.

While the costs for these services can be calculated, there is no possible way to assess the cost of pain, suffering, loss of a loved one, early death, the loss of quality life, and other priceless factors. Many individuals are caught up in the web of deceit that has been spun by The House of Deception (HOD) over the past half century.

The concept of "Who Stole My Food" gives rise to many questions: Who did it? Why did they do it? When did they do it? How did they do it? What did they do?

In this book, I declare the answers to these questions from my perspective as a Food Scientist and Nutritionist. I believe those individuals who would like to be healthy throughout their life can do so by following the simple guidelines provided in this Series.

This book is written for all people, including the poor as well as the wealthy! No One, **No, Not One,** is so poor that they cannot afford to be healthy. However, I do know of many individuals who cannot afford to be sick.

"Health is like money, we never have a true idea of its value until we lose it." ~Josh Billings

Basic Assumptions

1. Cholesterol and animal fats are good for you!

This assumption is based largely upon the writings of Dr. Uffe Ravnskov, M.D. Ph.D., who is a nephrologist, but more than that, he is an exceedingly competent scientist, capable of a comprehensive, honest, critical review of all the literature dealing with cholesterol and animal fats, as related to coronary heart disease.
This he did in his book "The Cholesterol.Myths" which was first published in 1991. (38) **In this book he clearly dissected the publications from**

the HOD, exposing their lies and manipulation of data to support their agenda. (*A must read*)

2. The fat and cholesterol idea is a diversion from a much greater deception.

The fact that the fat-cholesterol idea is pure myth, as disclosed by Dr. Ravnskov, this is but the tip of the "Iceberg." The nine myths are but a mere distraction from a much greater deception that has been causal for hundreds of chronic diseases, affecting millions of people during the past half century. Under the guise of avoiding CHD by avoiding animal fat and cholesterol containing foods, the HOD has very cleverly deprived humans of their ability to build and maintain the very support structure of the body, thus giving rise to many chronic diseases which I refer to as Connective Tissue Disorder (CTD).

3. Genetic Repair

By its very nature, the body is prepared through genetic programming, to manufacture and repair all of the various organs, tissues, and the chemicals needed for complete metabolism. This would include enzymes, hormones, proteins, fats, carbohydrates, antibodies, co-factors, plus many more. That is, provided that the body has received the nutritional elements required, in a timely ongoing manner, for the building and maintenance of the body. This is equally essential during fetal development, as well as after birth and throughout life.

4. Species Nutritional Differences

The differences between the nutritional needs of humans and other animals as to their actual chemical needs are quite small. Since the early 1960s, I perceive a concerted effort on the part of the HOD to distance human nutrition from animal nutrition.

5. Disease and Malnutrition

Most non-infectious, chronic diseases are the result of malnutrition — an excess, or lack of, the nutritional factors such as vitamins, minerals, trace minerals, amino acids, fatty acids, crude fiber, protein and carbohydrates in the diet. With complete and balanced nutrition, the body is far more likely to be able to fight off many of the infectious diseases.

Why do you think the infectious diseases represent higher risks for the very young and the elderly? It is because they are the most likely to be malnourished!

6. Know Your Source on Nutritional Information—is it truthful?

All of the information on health and nutrition, irrespective of its source, is suspect and should be critically examined to ensure its truthfulness, and that it passes the common sense analysis.

7. Foods — Good or Bad?

There are no bad foods but eggs are the best, with milk, pork and beef being better than most other foods. We do need a wide variety of foods, including fruits, vegetables, and cereal products, all in moderation.

8. Do You Need a Supplement?

A good RDA based vitamin and mineral supplement is a *must have* in the diet, if only to ensure that you will not be lacking any of the trace minerals that are so essential to good health.

9. There are no half truths!

When infomercials, news releases on TV, the radio, newspapers or magazines are being considered, please remember, there is no such thing as a half-truth. ***Anything less than the whole truth is a lie!*** One cannot be slightly pregnant any more than one can be a semi-virgin!

"But let your conversation be, Yea, yea; Nay, nay: for whatever is more than these, cometh of evil" (Matt. 5:37 KJV)

10. When is Nutrition Helpful?

Unless you are dead, it is never too late to improve your health through good nutrition.

Introduction

This book is not a book ***of*** medicine, but rather a book ***about*** medicine — the good and the bad of medical practices and policies ***as I perceive them***. It is a book written as a lay person for lay people. I am not a physician, but rather a food scientist and nutritionist. The book has been a labor of love over the past five years. Prior to that, I spent about seven and one-half (7 ½) years at the University Of Missouri and Michigan State University, where I earned my Doctorate in Food Science and Nutrition in 1961. This was followed by twenty years in the Food Industry, with three major corporations, where I conducted and/or directed numerous primarily applied research projects.

My work covered the areas of Product Development, Quality Assurance and Sanitation, with a very wide range of different food ingredients in virtually all types of foods, including pet foods. For eight years I was involved in nutritional studies confirming the adequacy of RDA type formulations, to provide Complete and Balanced Nutrition for dogs and cats. These studies included multiple breeds, and all life cycles through more than three generations of each breed tested.

I took early retirement in 1981, and have remained active in a variety of business interests, as well as starting to write this book five years ago. I see the writing of this book as my life mission, and as I reflect on all of life's experiences, the formal education, the work experiences in foods, nutrition and health. — I am satisfied that there is a purpose in everything we do in life. Though I have known most of the information contained in this book for many years, I did not comprehend the significance of that knowledge. I believe that a much higher power has provided the inspiration for me to pull these scientific facts together in a manner that can be comprehended and utilized by anyone who takes the time to read it.

Where possible, I have attempted to sprinkle common sense as a seasoning while writing this series of books on health and nutrition, so that you may see more clearly how ridiculous are the recommendations of the HOD. There is so much misinformation about health, diets, vitamins, minerals, herbal products, natural, organic, chemicals, naturopathy, homeopathy, holistic cures, antioxidants, good foods, bad foods., weight management programs etc., etc. that most people do not know what to believe or not believe.

I believe you will gain the greatest benefit from reading this book by first laying aside all information you may have regarding any particular foods, veganism, vegetarianism, nutrition, vitamins, organic foods versus natural foods, proteins, antioxidants, fats, carbohydrates, vitamins, minerals, fiber, weight management, etc. If you are not interrupting yourself with questions as you read through it, you are much more likely to understand the messages included in this book. I would then ask you to reread it to see if there are any unanswered questions.

Prior to reading this book, I suggest that, for a clearer understanding of the position that I take with respect to those in the HOD, you review two, three, or more of these references: (1,2,3,4,5,6,8,9,11,12,13,15,16,17,19,20,21,23,25, 26,27,28,29,30,31,33,34,35,36,41,43,44,45,46,47,48 ,49)).

You can review any you choose, and choose as many as you want, to satisfy yourself that what I am telling you is true.

About five years ago, I was reflecting upon many of my life experiences, including growing up around animals, working in a grocery store in the Midwest, my formal education in Food Science & Nutrition, and twenty years conducting research. in the food industry. It was at this time that I decided that I could, with my background, help some of those individuals who were overweight to lose some weight safely, and <u>keep</u> it off, applying the principals that I had learned.

In the process of writing this book, I realized I could not fit all of the important puzzle pieces that complete the picture of good health. into one book. Therefore, I will be telling the full story in a series of books as follows:

Book I "Who Stole my Food"
Tells the truth about deceptive recommendations and why we may be causing our own chronic diseases by following these half truths and myths.

As we add to the coffers of our caregivers, this book gives sound reasons why keeping you healthy is not the motive of the HOD.

Book II "Achieving A More Perfect Health"
Provides the philosophy necessary to ensure that you can achieve good baseline nutrition. In so doing, prevent the majority of non-infectious chronic diseases that steal the quality of life from millions of people today.

Book III "The Miracle of Eggs"
Compares various foods to eggs, (the best food in the world) and discloses the significant differences that would allow a person to ensure their dietary needs are met based upon the best choices in selection of their foods.

Nutrition is about health, not about medicine and, conversely, medicine is not about nutrition!

Good baseline nutrition begins with having all of the nutrients in the diet that are required for good health.. Only a few of the chemicals needed by humans, or other animal species, are in the foods that we eat or the supplements that one might take. The body has a rather large and complex factory where many other chemicals are produced, *provided the basic raw materials are present for the factory to operate successfully.*

In a word, all of the essential chemicals must be present for the diet to be ***complete.*** These needs have been known for a half century, and have been fully tested with the domestic farm animals where there is a financial motivation for the animals to be healthy. The financial motivation for your good health is not present for those working in the HOD. Indeed, they would likely lose seventy-five percent (75%) of their business if their patients could avoid most of the chronic diseases through better nutrition. Their financial interest is best served if you are unhealthy!

The second important factor is that one must have the proper amount of each of the required chemicals for the diet to be **balanced.** It is, in many ways, like trying to bake a cake where one must have all of the ingredients. But it is exceedingly important to have the right amount of each ingredient as well — one must have both to be successful. Additionally, the recipe must include the proper sequence for mixing the ingredients and the proper temperature and time for cooking, or you can get a flop!

So it is with having your factory supplied with all of the essentials, in the proper amount, at the right time, for it to produce the numerous chemicals that it must produce if you are to truly be healthy. There are numerous enzymes, co-enzymes, hormones, catalysts, blood cells, muscle cells, nerve cells, bone cells. etc., that your body is programmed to build and maintain. This is essential for replacement of the cells of the body, should those cells be damaged in accidents, or as they wear out with age. That is, if one is to sustain good health..

When some of these chemicals are missing, or are not there at the right time, the body may try to substitute another chemical. Much of the time, it just cannot produce all that is needed for each of the functions due to non-availability of nutrients at the time needed. It has been estimated that the normal body is likely to perform a billion chemical reactions each day within your factory. Of course, there are several other bodily functions that must be coordinated or performed to achieve the full benefit of having a complete and balanced diet. These include exercise, sleep, and waste elimination, to name but a few. This is discussed in Book II of this Series. The main point is that achieving good base line nutrition begins with having a diet that is ***complete and balanced***.

This book is being written primarily for the lay people interested in protecting their health. to the fullest, based upon current scientific knowledge; and secondarily, for the various health professionals who attended college subsequent to 1965. These individuals may work within the HOD, not realizing that their education, if it included nutrition, was not based upon the truth.

I would like to emphasize the word knowledge, which is quite different from information. We all have an abundance of information on health and nutrition; however, unless the information is based on truth, it simply does not constitute knowledge!

The very fact that the information is reported in the most prestigious medical journals or from the most respected government laboratories, agencies, or research foundations does not make it true. For instance, in the late 1950s we were advised by the American Heart Association (AHA) that we should eat no more than one egg a week, but throw the yolk away. Their position now, forty years later, is that it is safe to eat one egg per day, including the yolk.

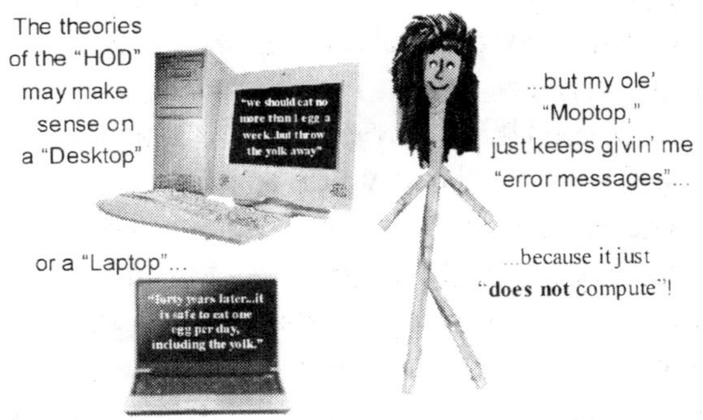
The theories
of the "HOD"
may make
sense on
a "Desktop"
"we should eat no more than 1 egg a week..but throw the yolk away"
or a "Laptop"...
"forty years later...it is safe to eat one egg per day, including the yolk."
...but my ole'
"Moptop,"
just keeps givin' me
"error messages"...
...because it just
"**does not** compute"!

I am totally unaware of any change in the chemistry of eggs over the past forty years. And to my knowledge, there has been no real change in the chemical needs of humans, or any of the domestic animals for that matter.

This is only one of many recommendations advanced by the HOD over the past half century that have been challenged by numerous independent scientists and physicians. It appears to me that these various recommendations have been advanced more to satisfy a profit/power agenda, rather than to helping people become healthier.

The basic concept that I hope to communicate is that one should never lose sight of common sense. This includes the recommendations being made by anyone, including the HOD, as to what is good or bad for your health.. All too often, the money trail is obvious; however, there are many instances where the lies are not easily discerned. This is especially true when they are repeated numerous times by the well recognized and respected members, which I include in my definition of the HOD. By design, they speak with "one voice" — but whose voice is it?

The advent of the food pyramid and the scheme to recommend elimination of animal fats and cholesterol containing foods from the diets of humans has been very detrimental to the health. of most Americans. These recommendations, by my estimates, have been the cause of more than seventy five percent of the chronic diseases seen over the past half century.

Over time with the animal rights groups objecting to any form of animal testing, a new form of research testing became popular. This was based upon the use of double blind studies including placebos.

However, in the experimental design of the studies, they ignored the need for much of the standardizations that had been meticulously followed in earlier studies, and the experiments did not search for the truth, but rather for the answer the researcher wanted. With this approach to research many of the research studies reported results that could not be confirmed by independent scientists, who were searching for the truth. When such studies cannot be legitimately confirmed, this is usually referred to as "junk science". This type of "research" is causal in the almost daily announcements in the news media, as well as scientific publications, where something is good for you today, but bad for you tomorrow.

I believe that this has been the case with the animal fat/cholesterol theory with respect to these chemicals being causal in coronary heart disease., strokes and hardening of the arteries.

At this time, it appears almost everything is given to sound bites and spin, in pursuit of money and power — the truth just doesn't seem to matter — even when you're very life is at stake.

It was not too long before the end of WWII that penicillin was developed, and was considered the miracle drug — which it was. Over the years, many antibiotics and vaccines were found to control and/or prevent such infectious diseases as small pox, polio, measles, pneumonia, anthrax, tuberculosis, diphtheria, typhoid, etc. This was a real boon for individuals, and no doubt saved many lives.

However, it may have been viewed as a two edged sword for the HOD. Were they putting themselves out of business? Perhaps the HOD would be better described as "The House of

Darkness." It appears evil to me for those individuals to submit and perpetuate the lies that have been causal in so many deaths, so much pain and suffering. Those lies are also causal in financial ruin through the use of fear tactics, supported by junk science designed to provide the answers they want, rather than searching for the truth.

If their recommendations are not directed toward the growth and profitability of their business at the expense of the patient's good health and well being, then I have to believe their recommendations are due to ignorance. In either instance, this madness should stop now!

Chapter 1

The House of Deception (HOD)

A "One Voice" Hoax — when the HOD controls the research grants and the most prestigious medical journals publishing the research results, this does not make those results true! It is but an attempt to convey creditability to their false claims as being supported by "the preponderance of research".

To be sure, **the information contained in this book is my personal opinion,** and I am sure there will be those individuals and organizations that hold a different opinion on these matters that deal with health and nutrition.

While searching the literature on health and nutrition, I have observed several references to "The House of Medicine." What is not so apparent, is who or what does this include? In my endeavor to find the truth with respect to health and nutrition issues, there is ample evidence that recommendations have been made over the past fifty or sixty years which are not, and could not be based upon the truth. These recommendations are often repeated by the vast majority of those individuals and institutions that are perceived as authorities in matters of health and nutrition. The diverse group that I refer to represents a much bigger group than I would consider "The House of Medicine" to be, thus the need to call it by another name.

What I have observed to be happening over the past half century, suggests that the problem is getting much worse, and the pace of change is ever accelerating. I do not consider this to be a conspiracy, but more like an autocracy which has given rise to a "one voice" position from what I shall call: **"The House of Deception" (HOD)**, This "one voice" approach was taken to secure a greater degree of authority, prestige, and thus believability among the people of the world. This has resulted in uncontrolled escalation of the cost of medical care in this country by bringing about significant increases in the types and incidences of non-infectious, chronic diseases.

The "one voice" approach appears to have been very effective in that, clearly, most people interviewed expressed their concern regarding cholesterol, animal fat, eggs, beef, pork, and dairy products, as well as the concept that one can obtain the essential nutriments by following the recommendations provided in the food pyramids and the food guidelines.

Of the hundreds of organizations reviewed, I found only one that did not speak with the "one voice" approach to health. and nutrition.

Through control of research grants, (who gets published, and numerous other factors), is it any wonder that the "preponderance of evidence" usually referred to would make it more credible to most people. Little do the people realize the extent to which this "preponderance" is controlled, to ensure consistency, so that it is perceived as credible. A critical review of their research grants has shown the degree to which they have gone to deceive the people. The best example I have seen is in the disclosures to be found in Dr. Ravnskov's book, The Cholesterol.Myths. It is like the political talking points, where the objective is to repeat the same thing by multiple individuals so often that it is believed to be credible, never questioning if it is the truth!

I am providing here but a partial list of the organizations reviewed, that perpetuate these erroneous recommendations in most of their publications.

The American Heart Association (AHA), The American Medical Association (AMA), The American Cancer Society (ACS), The United States Department of Agriculture (USDA), The Food and Drug Administration (FDA), National Institutes of Health (NIH), National Research Council (NRC), National Academy of Science (NAS), the Communicable Disease and Prevention Centers (CDC), the pharmaceutical industry, the food processing industry, the supplement industry, plus a number of trade organizations, and many of the major medical facilities. To this day, they tell the same lies, and after almost sixty years, most people believe them.

There are many innocent individual professionals caught up in this war. These include some physicians, dieticians and scientists, within the above named organizations. They are probably there due to job security issues and some are probably there because they actually believe what has been published over the past sixty years by the above well respected groups. Not all supplement manufacturers or food companies are considered part of the HOD.

None the less, any medical decisions you are required to make, at the very least, should be critically reviewed prior to taking medications or having a surgical procedure performed. Consider the consequences of any mistake, deception or ignorance on the part of the medical professionals in whose hands you all too often place your life. In every instance that I can conceive of, all of the benefits are to the person providing the care, treatment, diagnosis or surgery. Their mistakes or lack of knowledge provides more opportunity to diagnose, treat, or care for the patient, thus increasing the cost for medical care and services. The patient left with their mistakes, deceptions, or ignorance, is the big loser by either dying, or having to overcome the adverse effects of such treatments.

The agenda and profit motivation. appear to be true conflicts of interest with the good health. one has a right to expect. When going to a medical professional, whether it is a nurse's aid, LVN, RN, nurse practitioner, physician's assistant, physician or other types of professionals working within the HOD, you have the right to receive honest and competent professional help.

There are references in the literature that refer to a war on health that deals with the fight against diseases. This was directed primarily toward the infectious diseases such as malaria, small pox, typhoid, and many other diseases.

At this time I believe there is an ongoing war on health that has been underway for half a century. I am referring to the ***non-infectious, chronic diseases. For these diseases, the HOD generally claims the causes are unknown, there are no known cures, nor do they know any forms of prevention!*** About the only thing they seem to know or concern THEMSELVES with is diagnostics, treatment — (which may be with medications or surgeries.), care in hospitals, therapy or rest homes of various types. From the records on this battle field, it appears the patients are the enemy.

The majority of the population is, or has been, totally oblivious of this war! The battle field is strewn with millions of people who have died, or suffer the painful and expensive consequences of this long ongoing battle, not even knowing they have been caught up in this damnable war! The strategic plan of the HOD has been drafted with precision, and the tactics masterfully executed over the years. This was done by those that would like to have more business and profits, even if it is at the expense, pain and suffering of their patients, by creating a greater incidence of chronic diseases.

The strategic plan as I see it, along with the many tactics used, has out maneuvered the majority of individuals, giving rise to many of the chronic diseases experienced over the last fifty to sixty years. There has certainly been a significant increase in the **types** of different chronic diseases (at last count, more than a thousand), and most individuals, I believe, have observed a dramatic increase in the **incidence** of the various chronic diseases. This is not so much due to the improved diagnostic capabilities, but is more likely due to the recommendations that have been forthcoming from the HOD.

The medical professionals are certainly not all bad. They have made great strides in numerous areas of medicine. My primary concern is with the "one voice" position of the HOD, why it exists, and the manner in which it is sustained!

But, what is the "one voice" saying?

In their mission statements, they:

- talk about wanting people healthy
- want to find the cure, but it sounds like they mean treatment
- want to prevent diseases, but it sounds like they mean avoidance of diseases

Their recommendations reveal the:

- cause of disease is unknown
- cure is not possible
- prevention is for the future
- treatment is what you get — with medication or surgery
- absence of nutrition from their thinking / understanding
- use of fear tactics to sell their services

- genetic factors probably cause all matters unknown to them
- facts regarding risk factors for disease, are but suppositions

In my search of the literature, the "one voice" never speaks of nutrition as a possible causal factor for the chronic diseases. Other than, a casual mention at times, that diet may be a factor, but it is almost never given credence. This is clearly evidenced by the fact that virtually none of their research grants have any connection what so ever with nutrition. They speak only of diet, as eating a heart healthy diet, by avoiding animal fats cholesterol, beef, pork, eggs and, of course, discouraging the use of a good RDA type vitamin and mineral supplement.

I have never found any reference that suggests any link with the various types of cancers, neurological diseases, circulatory diseases, Arthritis, pulmonary diseases, or any of the other chronic diseases, as being related to nutritional deficiencies. Only their risk factors of animal fats, cholesterol, and smoking or second hand smoke! Wouldn't it be wonderful if someone actually investigated the nutritional relationship to the chronic diseases, and much better yet, if a simple thing, like **good baseline nutrition,** were found to **prevent** these diseases? Good baseline nutrition will never be achieved if one is following their recommendations!

My philosophy on this, and my reasons for what I believe, will be explained fully as you go through the book.

Are There Any Good Physicians?

Mere competence and good ethics does not make one a good physician! After all, you must be able to get in to see them in a reasonable period of time. I consider myself very fortunate that I have garnered a group of health.-care professionals in whom I have great confidence. Over time they have demonstrated their technical skills, ethics, and priorities. The health of my family is more important to them than the almighty dollar.

There are many health.-care professionals who are equally committed to their work.

I have known several physicians, as well as other professionals, who refuse to be a part of the system that wants them to perform numerous unnecessary diagnostic procedures, surgeries or to dispense medications that have numerous dangerous side effects. They have taken early retirements or established private practices. The scientists in this category find research grants virtually impossible to find, and even though they find private funds for their research, their findings are rarely published in any of the prestigious medical journals.

One of the reasons for writing this series of books on health and nutrition relates to a conversation I had about five years ago with a scientist who worked for The American Egg Board. This particular scientist had published an article on the nutritional values of various foods, and appeared to be ambivalent on the nutritional value of eggs. When I asked him what he thought the best food in the world was, he answered milk. When I questioned his decision, he said he meant the colostrum, or first milk after giving birth. I then reminded him of the simple fact that if you take a fertilized egg and incubate it for twenty–one days you have a healthy chicken that received 100% of its total nutritional needs from that egg. No other food in the world can equal that feat!

He then acknowledged that it wasn't that he disagreed with me on that, but that there was one thing that I had to understand. That was that he received all of his research funding from the U.S. Department of Agriculture. They review all scientific articles funded by them prior to publishing, and he had to be very careful about what he said!

With that, the red flag went up! They can't even tell the truth! I immediately started writing this book, because I would like the population to know the truth, rather than the lies that have been so damaging to the health of so many people over the past half century.

The problem as I see it is that medical professionals who are honest, conscientious, hard working, and compassionate, are fighting something that is a lot bigger than they are. Their job security, research grants, prestige, or any number of other factors are in jeopardy, should they disclose their true beliefs. The patient is most likely to be the one that suffers from these more dominant factors in the professional's life. Many of them speak with the "one voice" on matters dealing with health..

As a patient, one should be aware of this when deciding whether or not to follow their recommendations. Common sense should play an important part in your decision making, rather than accepting all that is said on blind faith.

There have been many miracles in medical practices, but when a physician resets and splints your broken leg so that the body can heal, if he or she is the one who tripped you, causing the broken leg in the first place, you would have difficulty giving accolades. Likewise, if you are given medication for pain control, and you have a major heart attack because of the side effects, then this is no miracle! There should be full disclosure of all known side effects.

It is equally unwarranted to recommend surgeries when they are not needed. Be very cautious when you have to make decisions with respect to medications or surgeries.

"The best and most efficient pharmacy is within your own system." ~Robert C. Peale

The Struggle: Health versus Wealth & Power

Initially, this book was to be called "The War on Health". In many respects, what I have learned over these past five years makes it appear a lot like war. The major problem is that most of the population doesn't realize what has been going on.

It is my opinion that the planning for this war could well have started following the formation of the World Medical Association in 1945-1947. The development of penicillin and other antibiotics for the control of infectious diseases was very successful. Perhaps so successful, that these developments gave rise to fear within the HOD that the population was becoming too healthy. The progress in identifying the vitamins, minerals, essential amino acids, essential fatty acids, and other nutritional factors were having great benefit to improved health. of humans, as well as the farm animals. After all, these developments were likely to stifle the growth and profitability of the medical industry. They really couldn't play games with the farm animals because these animals are grown for profit. Any successful farmer has a financial motive for his or her animals to be healthy. There is no such financial motivation for the doctor if you are healthy — just the opposite! If you are healthy, there is far less need for his or her services.

The declaration in the late 1950s that animal fats and cholesterol in the diet were killers, causal in coronary heart disease, hardening of the arteries and strokes, represented the beginning of the war.

It was also in this timeframe that the recommendation to take a multiple vitamin and mineral supplement was reversed. The USDA recommended that people should get all of their nutrition from their foods, based upon the food pyramid, instead.

A well coordinated effort by the HOD ensured that they spoke with "one voice" in bringing forth their recommendations about the primary causes and risk factors for chronic diseases. To be frank about it, these folks can't be trusted with your nutritional decisions

What the HOD would like you to believe:
(This is based upon thousands of articles published over the past fifty+ years.)

- Their interest is for you to be healthy.
- Physicians are knowledgeable in nutrition.
- Dietitians are knowledgeable in nutrition.
- High cholesterol is related to coronary heart disease, strokes and hardening of the arteries
- They are interested in prevention of chronic diseases.
- They are interested in cures for chronic diseases.
- Cholesterol and animal fats are bad for you.
- Meat (beef and pork) is bad for you
- Eggs are bad for you
- Milk and dairy products are bad for you.
- Eating to the food pyramid will provide for all of your nutritional needs
- Multiple vitamin/mineral supplements are not necessary for good health.

- Nutritional needs for humans are significantly different from other animal species.
- Vegetable oils should replace butter and other animal fats.
- Soy protein is a good replacement for meat, milk, and eggs.
- Fast-Foods are bad for you.
- Genetics are causal in many of the chronic diseases and genomic nutrition is the future to improving one's health. on an individualized basis.

There has been an ongoing effort to establish **lower standards** for many areas of the analytical guidelines that have been accepted for many years. The guidelines for any chronic disease are subject to change, at their whim, with or without benefit to health as has been seen with the cholesterol guidelines. I fear this is true with obesity, blood pressure, blood sugar and perhaps numerous other areas.
Each lowering of a standard or guideline creates more potential patients, giving cause for dispensing more medications or recommending more surgeries!

These new lower standards result in an ever increasing percentage of the population being declared at risk for numerous health problems:

- One-half the US Population has high cholesterol and is at risk of coronary heart disease, strokes, and hardening of the arteries — needing cholesterol lowering medications!

- Fifty percent (50%) of the population have been declared obese and another twenty five percent (25%) overweight.
- Hypertension (high blood pressure) standards are now in the process of being lowered from 170/90 to 100/60 – fifty million or more people are affected.
- Arthritis – more than 100 types — affecting seventy five million people.
- IBS — Irritable Bowel Syndrome — affects twenty percent (20%) of population (Sixty million people).
- There is increasing concern for Type II diabetes
- There is increasing concern for obesity with the primary solution being the recommendation for gastric bypass surgery rather than a safer, less expensive approach.

What is the impact of these recommendations and the various revised lower guidelines upon the health and well being of the U.S. Population? How will these changes affect the growth and profitability of the HOD?

Who is on the other side?

With blind faith, individuals who want to be healthy rely on the experts to be their guardian protectors in matters concerning health and nutrition. This might best be described as "the lambs being led to slaughter" or as some say, "the herd instinct". Fortunately, there are a number of very capable independent scientists and physicians who are on your side. However, their voices are often muted, and their research condemned by the concerted efforts of the named groups who represent the other side in this war.

The CDC records show that in spite of the billions of dollars spent on cancer research., and the significant and successful results of: removing smoke from the work place; lowering tar, and reducing consumption of tobacco products; the ever expanding types of scanning devices to spot cancer early; the development of numerous surgical techniques such as bone marrow transplants, etc., the war against cancer has been a losing proposition. They reported 193 deaths per 100,000 from cancer in 1950 and a total of 209 deaths per 100,000 in 2000! In that same fifty year period, they report only slight reductions in strokes and coronary heart disease., and even those reductions are in dispute.

The CDC has reported on the causes of some of the cancers, and each cancer may be caused by different things. In one instance an enzyme deficiency was believed to be the cause. When looking at the composition of that enzyme, it contained a vitamin that was probably lacking in the diet, and if so, would support the contention that malnutrition is causal in this form of cancer.

As a youngster growing up in the 1930s and 1940s, like most people, I was in awe when in the presence of physicians or registered nurses. Theirs was a noble cause — wasn't it? Today the picture has undergone dramatic change and the awe has been replaced with woe! In the evolutionary process of medicine, perhaps driven by competition or the need for profits, each change being made in medical care as relates to chronic diseases, appears to have been made to the detriment of the patient!

We now see nursing assistants or aids who can work the hospital floor with only three months training. We see LVNs, or volunteer workers, even the janitorial staff, providing assistance to patients because the assigned RN has been relegated to paper pushing administrative details. If they are busy elsewhere, attending to paper work, they are not available to attend to, and properly follow, the patient's condition. This makes it impossible to take immediate action when there is a critical change in condition.

With physicians, the changes have likewise been detrimental for the patients. We now have physician assistants, nurse practitioners, and rather than the standard M.D. of olden days, in some states, we find other types of medical training, such as osteopathy, using the M.D. as well. There are other areas of study that provide differing forms of training for the practice of medicine such as Naturopathy, Homeopathy, Holistic, etc. While this may be a good business decision to reduce the cost of the labor pool, it clearly does not benefit the patient to have a nurse's aid who is untrained to discern critical changes as they occur with some patients. Nor does it benefit the patient if they cannot communicate with the caregivers because the caregiver cannot understand, or be understood in, English. Then, when the patient's condition deteriorates, they can then arrange for the patient to go to the Intensive Care Unit (ICU) or Critical Care Unit (CCU). There, better care can be provided, along with the numerous scans, x-rays, etc. now available. The final cost will likely be triple what it would have been, had the problem been diagnosed and treated in a timely manner. My greatest sympathy goes to those physicians and registered nurses whose careers have been seriously compromised by the changes mentioned above.

The control appears to be out of the hands of the health professionals and into the hands of HMO's and/or health insurance companies. People untrained in medicine now tell the health professionals what they can or cannot do. In some instances it is the bean counters who order unnecessary diagnostic procedures or surgeries.. This reflects an out of control medical system. Who are they to decide what my medical needs are? The physicians and registered nurses are the ones trained to diagnose and treat medical problems — not some business graduate who knows how to make money at the expense of the patients.

The patient is the one to suffer when the educational standards are reduced to levels of gross incompetence. Where patient care is needed, the care must provide the confidence that the best that can be done, is indeed being done.

The HOD, on the other hand, while getting the benefits of lower labor costs, increases the costs incurred by patients. This is, at least partly, due to the lack of competence, and thus the need for ever more expensive hospital stays in ICU or CCU. That is, if the patient is lucky enough to survive whatever may have been lacking in their care, as a direct result of the caregivers lack of training for the job being performed.

This has certainly provided for a much greater level of employment of the lower income, less trained individuals. At the same time it has decimated the medical fields of endeavor. Additionally, these practices of cost cutting have been causal in the significant increase in post operative infections within the medical facilities. Infections caused by organisms such as streptococcus, meningitis, staphylococcus, and pneumonia, to name a few!

We the people deserve better than this from our medical professionals!

There have been many quotes throughout history regarding health. Here are but a few…

"Some remedies are worse than the disease."
Publilius Syrus(fl. B.C. 42)

"Doctors prescribe medicine of which they know little, to cure diseases of which they know less, in human beings of which they know nothing."
Voltaire (1694-1778)

"The prerequisite for today's medical policy is naturally the currently predominant system of medicine. The sick are the source of income, therefore it is necessary for sick people to be there; Yes, it proves advantageous if one makes the people artificially sick."
Dr. med. Steintl: 'International Medical Policy', 1938 Berlin

"Research is subordinated, (not to long-term social benefit) but to an immediate commercial profit. Currently, disease (not health) is one of the major sources of profit for the pharmaceutical industry, and the doctors are willing agents of those profits."
Dr. Pierre Bosquet, Nouvelle Critique, France, May 1961

"Every month, millions are in fact being damaged by treatment which is supposed to be helping them."
Dr. Werner Lehmpfuhl, general practitioner in Hanover, in the weekly magazine Welt am Sonntag, July 29, 1973

Chapter 2

The Trickery of the Food Pyramids

(Trickery: "The practice of crafty underhanded ingenuity to deceive or cheat" as defined by Merriam Webster)

Who stole my food? Who stole my eggs, milk, beef, pork, and told me that I no longer need to take a multi vitamin and mineral supplement based upon the Recommended Daily Allowance (RDAs)? It was those individuals who speak with "one voice." Some refer to them as "The House of Medicine" but I call them "The House of Deception (HOD).

The premise of this book is to declare that for a half century, the food pyramids and the food guidelines have been manipulated to deprive you of the best foods for good health.. The controlling factor in what I refer to as the HOD, has made recommendations under the guise of telling people how to be healthy.

Their recommendations serve just the opposite purpose, virtually stealing the best foods from the diets of humans. This causes numerous chronic diseases with their associated pain, suffering, and even premature death. This comes with a devastating price tag to the patients, and their families, while contributing an added tax burden, as required by the government, to pay for the increasing medical costs.

Plants versus Animals

In the beginning, the early scientists recognized the need to classify various things into groups. They called the individual elements found in the universe **inorganic** minerals. These included, but are not limited to, hydrogen, oxygen, iron, sodium, sulfur, potassium, gold, copper, etc. These represent a few of the minerals and trace minerals critical to many of the chemical reactions that promote essential metabolic processes. The total number of elements identified is ever changing. Many of the known elements are essential to have good health, while many are known to be highly toxic to man and animals. The benefit to health from all of the elements has yet to be determined. These included hydrogen, oxygen, iron, sodium, potassium, gold, copper and in all, the number stands at about 250 elements. The chemicals that contained carbon were classified as **organic** material that is found in living matter. They chose to classify the living matter into two groups, **plants** and **animals**. If it is alive in this universe, it will be one or the other. This classification has absolutely nothing to do with religion, or how the various animals, including humans, came into being. The use of the term animal, be it domestic farm animals, such as cows, pigs, sheep, chickens, turkeys; or domestic pets, such as dogs, cats, birds or fish; or humans, is because all of them are classified as animals. There is no reason for this usage to be a stumbling block due to anyone's religious beliefs.

All animals share numerous characteristics, though there are also many differences. The main point that I want to make in comparing the nutritional needs of humans, domestic farm animals and domestic pets, is that once the foods consumed leave the stomach, or its equivalent, the chemicals found are very similar indeed. The chemical processes for the metabolic pathways that utilize these chemicals are basically the same; they have similar organs, having similar functions, such as liver, kidney, heart, bone, connective tissues, lungs, skin, reproductive organs, etc. Those animals that lay eggs do have different reproductive processes.

The nutritional needs of the various species of animals, based upon the Recommended Daily Allowances (RDAs), differ primarily in the amount of each chemical needed, due to the size and/or the age of the animal. The various species of animals (domestic farm animals and domestic pets) that I am comparing to humans served as the test animals for early nutrition studies prior to the early 1960s.

Once the theories were confirmed with the smaller animals, they were tested and confirmed with humans. It was in the early 1960s that testing procedures were changed drastically. It was also at this time that the HOD saw a need to distance human nutrition from that of the domesticated animals, and de-emphasized the need for medical students to study the science of nutrition.

There are many individuals who are absolutely confused by the frequent reports in the medical journals, television news reports, and other media sources that report one thing today, and the opposite the next, with respect to what a person should be doing to be healthy. For the most part, because of the esteem in which those in the HOD are held, due to their prestigious institutions and professional publications, the independent scientist can rarely have his or her voice heard. Should they be so lucky as to have their work published, they are immediately targeted by the HOD and declared to be crackpots.

The most damaging and erroneous recommendations made were:

- Avoid animal fats
- Avoid foods that contain cholesterol
- Eat to the food pyramid and follow the food guidelines
- Discourage the use of an RDA type supplement
- No more than one egg per week, but throw the yolk away
- Avoid beef, pork, and lamb
- Drink only non-fat or low fat milk
- Trim all of the visible fat from meats
- Chicken and turkey are better for your health.
- Soy protein is better for your health.
- Vegetable oils are better for your health.

Some of these recommendations were in place for more than thirty years, and caused massive financial losses to the beef, pork, egg and dairy industries. During the last five to ten years, there have been some changes in their positions;

however, their condemnation of these foods is not much improved to this day. According to the HOD, it is now safe to eat eggs provided you consume no more than 300 mg of cholesterol per day. One egg contains 220 mg cholesterol, and this recommendation would virtually eliminate meat and milk from the diet, even if you eat only one egg per day, and trim all visible fat from the very small portion of meat that would be allowed. And, of course, this would require a small serving of nonfat or very low fat milk, or none at all.

Avoid Animal Fats

Humans are animals, not vegetables! So what is wrong with eating animal fats? For forty years the main theme of the HOD was to avoid animal fats.

Even though some of the research that has been published during the last ten years has finally brought to light the fact that animal fats are not nearly as bad as had earlier been claimed, a large part of the population, and many of those in the HOD, continue to believe and declare that animal fats are bad for you. The only place that I have found a recommendation for the consumption of modest amounts of animal fats and a vitamin/mineral supplement has been on the web page for the Arthritis Foundation.(3) Indeed, the use of vegetable oils has been found to have some real health problems after all. These include trans fats, omega 6 versus omega 3 fatty acids, etc. Fats serve many functions in the human body, not the least of which is to provide insulation for temperature control, lubricity, and slickness for virtually every cell of the body. Fats also provide pliability or suppleness to virtually all tissues, such as the lungs, digestive tract, arteries (inside and out), nerve insulators, the joints, and the skin.

The greatest theft of all —
"Avoid Foods That Contain Cholesterol.

This one recommendation has probably dealt more pain and suffering to the human population than all others combined. It is clear to me that this was indeed a very clever move by the HOD. In one fell swoop they virtually eliminated the best foods in the world, saying that it was important for your heart health. to help prevent heart attacks, strokes and hardening of the arteries. This was a mere smoke screen for their real purpose, which set the stage for the human population to experience hundreds of chronic diseases affecting millions of people, due to the nutritional deficiencies caused by not eating the good foods that were stolen from your diet!

In my opinion, it has been done for money, power and sustained control — of your health.!

The very support structure of the body is dependent on the diet to provide an abundant source of amino acids that are more commonly found in animal tissues. These amino acids, proline, lysine, and glycine, plus the albumins found in milk and eggs, are used in the building and repair of the connective tissues. The proteins of the connective tissues, collagen and elastin, are found in every cell of the body along with cholesterol, and represent twenty five percent (25%) of the proteins found in the body.

Eat to the Food Pyramid and follow the Food Guidelines as recommended by the USDA.

Various surveys have been conducted by the USDA to determine the level of adherence to their recommendations by the general population. The survey results showed that 65-85% of the population does not conform to the guidelines. This certainly confirms that a very large segment of the population is poorly nourished — if the pyramid is valid. They make it appear as though they have "fine-tuned" the nutritional needs for humans, by having people count calories, grams of fat, protein, carbohydrates, fiber; select the types and amounts of sugars, fats, and various other items.

When I reflect back over the last fifty years, I sense that the human population is far worse off now than we were then. Many independent scientists, including myself, consider the food pyramid and the new food guidelines 2005 to be nothing more than "junk science". Clearly, seventy five (75%) of the population would benefit from taking a multi vitamin/mineral (RDA type) supplement, if for nothing more than to provide an inexpensive insurance policy — to ensure they are getting the trace minerals and vitamins needed in their diet!

Discourage the use of an RDA type supplement

Most of those individuals who speak with one voice assure us that we do not need the multi vitamin and mineral supplements when eating to the food pyramid. The trace minerals are my greatest concern since we now consume foods from all parts of the world. Many of the soils are often missing some of these elements, such as iodine, iron, fluoride, copper, etc. The farmers do not always fortify their soils due to costs, or perhaps, a simple lack of knowledge. So why should you and I take this risk when complete, safe supplements are available for less than a dime a day per person?

No more than one egg per week, but throw the yolk away!

The American Heart Association, along with many of the other associations, government laboratories and health related agencies set this recommendation in the late 1950s, allegedly due to the fat and cholesterol content. In my opinion, eggs are the best food in the world. In Book III of this series I compare various foods to eggs, so that you will realize the significant role that eggs should play in your diet. For more than five years now, I have consumed an average of 3+ eggs per day (2-6) and my cholesterol runs about 135 mg total. I attribute the balance in my diet, plus vitamin/mineral supplements, with other good foods like beef, pork, milk and some fruits and vegetables, as the primary cause for my good health. I recommend two to three whole eggs per day as part of a good diet.

Avoid Beef, Pork, and Lamb

Beginning in the mid 1950s the beef, pork, and lamb industry fell on hard times due to the controversy over animal fats and cholesterol. It was not until about 1990 that the American Heart Association finally declared that they thought it was now safe to eat beef or pork, in moderation, if it was trimmed of all visible fat. What many people do not realize is that the fat cells being contained in connective tissues are very important in supplying the chemicals necessary to maintain the body's support structure. These chemicals — proline, lysine, and glycine — along with the albumins, are found predominantly in animal tissues, milk, and eggs. They provide the basis for building and repairing the collagen and elastin. These protein sources are essential for every cell of the body, along with cholesterol and other animal fats.

I studied the connective tissues from various species, including chicken, turkey, beef, and pork in the mid 1960s. What I found was that chicken and turkey contained very little collagen or elastin, and what little it had, was of poor quality compared to pork or beef. This makes a lot of sense when you consider the size of the animals. The larger the animal, the stronger the connective tissues must be to support the larger organs. Pigs are more nearly the size of humans, and it follows that pig collagen is routinely used in the manufacture of stents that are used to repair arteries in humans. I believe that if more beef and pork were consumed, and less chicken and turkey, we would experience less of the chronic diseases that relate to weakness of bones, arteries, the digestive system, the nervous system, the skin, muscles and many others that will be reviewed in a later chapter.

Drink only non-fat or low fat milk

Milk is one of the better foods due to the minerals, amino acids and the fats present. The more recent research has shown that butterfat is indeed better for one's health than many vegetable oils. The best references that I can suggest is the work of Dr. Mary Enig and Sally Fallon, who have been the leading researchers on the fat controversy that started in the mid 1950's. They also were responsible for finding the trans fat / omega 6 problems, and the benefits of omega 3 fatty acids. Their early work is readily available on the internet under "The Oiling of America". (22)

Recommending Chicken and Turkey

The "one voice" recommendation to eat more chicken and turkey, instead of beef and pork, has been the practice in this country, as evidenced by the ever increasing production of chicken and turkey over the past fifty years. Indeed, *poultry meat* has largely replaced the *meat* (beef and pork) in most sausage products or other prepared foods. Recent production records report that 9.5 billion broiler chickens alone are produced each year in the U.S. Without question, it is easier and less expensive to produce a pound of chicken or turkey than beef or pork. Their usual recommendation is to remove the skin as well as all visible fat. In so doing, you are being deprived of even the very little, low quality connective tissue that is present in chicken or turkey, to your detriment. I am not saying that chicken or turkey are bad or unhealthful, simply that beef or pork are much better when it comes to their relative content of the chemicals necessary to help maintain one's connective tissues, such as collagen and elastin.

In my opinion, to deny your body the benefits to be gained by eating beef and pork, or sausages made from these meats, is likely to result in the unwanted deterioration of the support structure of the body such as bone, arteries, nerve insulators, cell walls, and factors affecting every cell of the body.

Recommending Soy Protein

Protein products from numerous sources have been recommended to ensure an adequate diet. It appears that many individuals have the belief that protein is protein, and it is of equal value, no matter its source. In fact, we would be much more accurate if we look at the Protein Efficiency Ratio (PER). With this type of rating system, eggs get the highest rating of 94, meaning that due to the balance of amino acids, 94% of egg protein is utilized by the body. Milk, meats, and fish score in the high 80s to the low 90s. Vegetable proteins such as soy proteins score 74. While it is true that by blending various protein sources one can produce a blend that would contain complete proteins, meaning that they contain all of the essential amino acids. There will still be many differences in composition, such as the types and amounts of fats, fatty acids, trace minerals, etc. These will contribute to a foods nutritional value. This makes it difficult to measure the *real* nutritional value when comparing foods. This will be reviewed in greater detail in Book III of this series.

Recommending Vegetable Oils

The vegetable oil/animal fat controversy has been on going for at least fifty (50) years. There are many different types of fats and fatty acids in the human body that are essential to maintaining good health.. Common sense should tell us that as animals, we should expect to maintain animal fats in our bodies.

Bone Composition and Structure.

The cartilage between the joints and the bones contain a base matrix of connective tissue which is collagen and elastin, which is subsequently mineralized. The soft bones have less of these minerals, primarily calcium, phosphorous, and magnesium, which serves to strengthen the bones. This involves vitamins such as Vitamins A, C, D, and E. Vitamin D is crucial and must be in a proper balance with the calcium and phosphorus. An excess of phosphorous to calcium can result in removal of calcium from the bones, weakening the bones, rather than strengthening them. Is that because the calcium has been withdrawn, or is it because the collagen, which gave the bone support in the first place, has been depleted or deteriorated to the point that crippling occurs?

One of the very confusing things that I have encountered in recent years has been the new proposed changes by the FDA and the USDA. To understand my point, I must provide some background information.

Since the mid 1950s animal feeds have been based upon a calcium / phosphorus ratio of 1.25:1. The RDAs issued in 1968 and 1980 were recommended by the NAS/NRC of the NIH. I have little or no faith in the various forms of the RDAs recommended subsequent to 1980. They now have numerous other recommendations like the RDIs (Recommended Daily Intake) and the safe upper limits of chemicals, etc. I am more concerned as to their agenda or motivation when considering their newer recommendations.

Only recently, the FDA proposed changing the calcium to phosphorus ratio from 1.25:1 to 1:1! This could lead to weakening of the bones by causing the removal of calcium, rather than deposition, which should increase bone density. In a later proposal the USDA proposed the ratio be 0.75:1.0, even worse for good bone health. What could be their purpose for such proposals? To better understand my concern, you need to be aware of other changes approved by the USDA and supported by the FDA since the early 1960s.

Since the mid 1960s a patented process used in the manufacture of gelatin from connective tissues involved the use of sodium hexa meta phosphate in dilute solution. This chemical causes connective tissues to absorb water, thus swelling the connective tissues. This same principle was then applied to the manufacture of processed meats, on the basis that the finished product would be juicier than conventional dry ham and bacon.

While this was true, it did increase the phosphates in the diet. This is why most hams are labeled as "water added" and also why one finds a lot of excess liquid upon opening the package. More recently I observed a frozen meat product in the grocery that was labeled on the front of the package "contains 30% added solution" and looking at the back of the label it disclosed the solution was a dilute sodium hexa meta phosphate solution. I see nothing wrong with this, except that it can increase the phosphates in the diet creating the need for more calcium, to maintain a proper ratio.

Yet another example of questionable recommendations from the FDA, USDA and AMA deals with folic acid supplementation. In 1948 it was recognized that folic acid was essential in the diet to prevent still births, neural tube defect or spina bifida in the new born infants. In the late 1950s these organizations were advising that we did not need multiple vitamin/mineral supplements, but rather, should eat to the Food Pyramid. This was changed in 1992, with the FDA recommending that women contemplating pregnancy should take a folic acid supplement of 400 mcg prior to conception and through pregnancy. Folic acid is reported to be the most common vitamin deficiency in humans. This deficiency results in a number of still births or infants with major disabilities, up to total loss of control of motor skills and control of bladder or bowel function. The CDC reported that in 2000 there were 20,000 or more such individuals being cared for in the U.S. at an annual cost of 200 million dollars/year.

Having been raised in the bible belt, I can't help but wonder what hurt those thirty years from 1960-90 must have brought to those families losing their children or having such deformed children. They were most likely blaming themselves or God for their misfortune, while they more nearly should have been blaming those organizations making those recommendations!

This was probably an honest mistake with their belief that adequate folic acid could be supplied with the foods recommended. Research conducted in Europe in the 1980s revealed that folic acid via supplements was more biologically available than that contained in the foods. As a result, most humans were reported to be receiving only half of their daily needs for folic acid. The low risk of taking an RDA type supplement during the years from 1960 through 1992, had that been their recommendation, could have significantly reduced the incidence of neural tube defect or spina bifida during these years.

The literature suggests the RDAs were developed with sufficient safety limits that a person could take up to three RDA based supplements a day with very low risk. Why then, did the FDA recently propose reducing their recommendations for folic acid from 400 mcg to 300 mcg a day? Are we not having enough defective births to satisfy them?

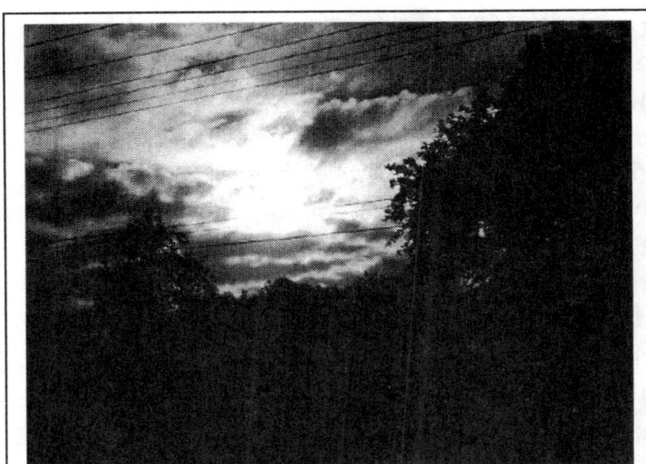

Pierced by the light of truth — every Deception shrouded in Darkness will be shattered

The Deceptions

Controlling the message on health

Through a concerted effort on the part of those who constitute the HOD, the system was established to help ensure that anyone in that group was on the same page so to speak, and providing the same information as to what is important in health.. Issues such as: animal fats and cholesterol are bad for you; therefore, don't eat beef, pork, milk, and no more than one egg per week, and then eat only the whites and throw the yolk away.

These recommendations started in the late 1950s, and as positions have changed, one continues to get only one voice. They now advise that in moderation, it is safe to drink low fat milk, eat beef or pork if lean and trimmed of visible fat, and one can now safely eat one egg per day, including the yolk. This "one voice" position from the HOD appears to have been believed by a majority of individuals as though it were equal to the Ten Commandments.

The HOD has, due to their recommendations, been causal in thousands of premature deaths, thousands of malformed infants and much of the chronic diseases in the U.S. and around the world along with the associated pain, suffering, premature loss of life and/or loved ones. This does not include the tremendous increase in the cost of medical treatments and health insurance which seem to know no limit.

One example to make the point, and there are probably many more that could be made, is the recommendation that was changed in the late 1950s from recommending that people take a vitamin and mineral supplement, to encouraging them not to take the supplement, but rather eat according to the food pyramid to ensure good health.. As early as the late 1940s the need for 400 mcg of folic acid on a daily basis was known.

Elimination of nutrition from the educational requirements

Nutrition in my opinion is a basic science and one that has all to do with sustaining good health.. In the early 1960s a number of changes were made to marginalize its importance in the HOD. It was in this time frame that human nutrition was isolated from animal nutrition even though the biological and chemical reactions occurring in all animals are very similar. The foods and the digestive systems are quite different between the various species, but once the food is digested, the chemistry of what happens is very similar.

In talking with personnel at the University of California, Irvine, which has a respected medical school, I was astonished to learn the University does not teach a single course in nutrition. (After fifteen to twenty minutes on the phone with the Registrar in discussing their schedule of courses, it was finally admitted that indeed they do not offer a single course in nutrition. This was immediately followed up with the comment that nutrition is now included in a lot of different courses; e.g., a course in kidney function would include nutritional studies that pertain to the kidneys. By my analysis the pre-med students need to have more than fragmented nutrition — they need the whole picture! What more important foundation could there be for good health. than nutrition?

Altering the methods of experimental testing — Junk Science

Why can't we believe what we read in the news media, hear on the radio or see on television? It seems that almost every day one of these news sources announces that new research shows this or that is good for whatever. The very next day the opposite conclusion is presented based upon another study.

In my opinion, these controversial results are due to flawed experimental designs where the study was designed to achieve the desired answer or result, with total disregard for the truth. Truly, it doesn't take much of a scientist to devise a study that conforms to a double blind study with placebos. What is likely lacking in such studies is a proper randomization of test subjects taken from populations that represent the normal populations.

For instance, if the test subjects are all chosen randomly from one ethnic group who is known to be deficient in a particular vitamin or mineral, then one could certainly show efficacy/benefit, if the test material would replace the deficient chemical. On the other hand if the experimental design were to include the standardization of all test subjects for good base line nutrition prior to testing the drug, then the test material would likely show little or no benefit. Most of the research conducted prior to 1960 was based upon standardized test subjects who made it possible for other scientists to replicate such studies, giving rise to a growing understanding of what nutritional needs were and how to prevent chronic diseases.

Fear tactics

Fear is a much used tactic by the HOD to ensure the growth and profitability of their business. Let's face it, if a professional tells you that you are likely to have a stroke or heart attack if you don't take a medication, or without that medication or the recommended surgery, you are going to die, most people will do as recommended by the professional. There are just too many stories in the news media of those instances where medications have been found to be unnecessary and have been removed from the market because of side effects worse than the initial problem, had the problem been real in the first place. Likewise, there have been many reports of unnecessary heart by-pass surgeries being performed, and those involved with doing the surgeries having to sell their hospitals or other facilities. They rarely lose their license to practice or admit to any wrong doing, even though they are said to have paid multimillion dollar fines for their actions. Not too satisfying for the patient, or their family!

Denying the need for humans to use RDA based vitamin and mineral supplements.

Most of the vitamins and minerals essential for good health in the animal kingdom were isolated in the 1930-1960 timeframe. The Recommended Daily Allowance (RDA) for each species of animal, including humans, were based upon the vitamins, minerals, and trace minerals known at the time, to be essential to good health in the various animals. The farm animals have been fed supplemental rations since the mid 1940s and the result has been healthy, profitable animals. Commercially prepared foods for domestic pets — dogs, cats, birds and fish — have been formulated for complete and balanced nutrition since the mid 1970s. Vitamin and mineral supplements were commercially available for humans in the early to mid 1940s, and were recommended by the medical professionals. However, in the late 1950s this was reversed for humans. It was then recommended that we should not take a vitamin or mineral supplement, but rather, eat the right balance of foods as suggested with the food pyramid to provide all of our nutritional needs. A concept that was promoted by the USDA and others, including physicians, dietitians and almost any organizations associated in any way with health issues, collectively known as the HOD.

There are those who would contend there are major differences between the various animal species, and that humans should be viewed as a totally separate entity as far as nutritional needs are concerned. I will concede there are several differences, though in the bottom line analysis there is but one major difference. There is a difference in the types of food eaten and in the digestive systems of the various species, but when one looks at the actual chemicals entering the blood system following digestion; they are truly quite similar, as the total number of vitamins and minerals recommended are virtually the same for all animal species. The amount of each chemical required being more a function of the normal size, weight, and stage in the life cycle for the particular species under consideration. The major difference between humans and all other species of animals is **CHOICE.** Humans alone have the ability to choose what they want to eat, whereas farm animals and domestic pets receive what the owner chooses to provide them. The farm animals eat forage crops and receive a supplemental ration to balance the diet. With dogs and cats that are fed commercially prepared pet foods as there only diet, each and every bite is complete and balanced. This is not so with humans. There are any numbers of factors that influence the choices people make when selecting the foods they will eat.

Good foods like meat, milk and eggs have been demonized

So, why is this so important? I'll tell you why, so you can decide where the truth lies on these three great foods. As mentioned elsewhere in this book, seventy-five percent (75%) of the medical costs in the U.S. are due to the chronic diseases.

By the HOD recommending the total elimination of beef and pork from the diet for at least thirty years (1960-1990); as they have done with milk and eggs to discourage their consumption as well, they have, with one single round of their ammunition been able to paralyze their prey — you and I!

Since 1990 they have relaxed their position on these foods, but still recommend severely restricting the consumption based primarily on the fat and cholesterol myths. Thanks to scientist like Dr. Ravnskov and the group called "The Skeptics" as well as numerous independent scientists, physicians, dieticians and others, some very big holes have been blown into the massive wall of lies promulgated by the HOD.

"Dumbing Down" the qualifications required for all health professionals.

The greatest operating cost in medical facilities probably relates to labor, which in my opinion has given rise to the significant change in the quality of service provided by these facilities. One can train for as little as three months and become a nurses aid or other medical assistant, who can provide a presence, but sorely lacking in the training necessary to readily identify critical changes in a patient during a life threatening situation. The less experience required for a job, the lower the wages and the greater the labor pool becomes, and indeed, this practice has virtually decimated the nursing profession. Similar changes have caused many physicians to leave the profession. Changes are now underway to restore some of the loss by legally requiring fewer patients per RN. You can find nurse practitioners as well as physician assistants, each with significantly less training than an M.D., performing much of the work of an M.D. In several States Osteopaths can use the designation M.D. This branch of medicine requires less training than your typical M.D. As I recall, this use of the M.D. designation was only allowed if they would agree to write prescriptions! Does this indicate a strong influence by the pharmaceutical industry?

Three years ago, in a major Orange County, CA hospital, only one Registered Nurse was scheduled on each floor of the hospital. This work load, in effect, reduced the RN to an administrative position rather than that of a practicing nurse. As of January 2004, this was changed and one RN can only be responsible for 1 to 5 patients, depending on the nature of the patient's illness.

In many businesses, the first budget items to be cut to shore up profits are those items that do not contribute directly to profits such as safety, janitorial/sanitation, quality control/assurance and maintenance personnel. There is little doubt that post operation infections represent a great risk for patients and are causal in many deaths. But this comes at a terribly high cost to the patient in terms of pain, suffering, and the risk of death. This simply due to the delays caused by a slow response to adverse change in the patient's condition!

Discounting the importance of good nutrition

After reviewing thousands of articles on health and disease in many of the scientific journals, news paper editorials and listening to professionals within the HOD over the past several years, I have rarely, if ever, seen or heard any of them make a recommendation that one should take a good RDA type vitamin and mineral supplement when they speak of treatment(s) for any of the many chronic diseases. From their comments, one could conclude that: either they want to conceal the benefits to be gained from taking a good vitamin and mineral supplement, or they really know very little about the essential nature of these chemicals as they relate to good health and the prevention of many of the chronic diseases. This should not be too surprising since very few physicians have studied the science of nutrition since the early 1960s. Their comments, when asked the question of, "Why do you not concern yourself with the patient's or test subject's nutritional status, have generally been; "there is no money in nutrition!"

This too becomes understandable when you consider the fact that if they make the patient healthy through good nutritional practices, this would be in conflict with building a profitable business practice. Their concept of medicine appears to be confined to diagnostics, treatment, (to include medications and surgeries.) and care in a treatment facility. With respect to chronic diseases, you seldom hear the words prevention or cure!

Discounting the importance of good sanitation practices

The scientific community has known for years that post operative infections result in many deaths in the U. S. One writer claimed this to be the fourth (4th) leading cause of death in the U.S. Staphylococcus infections are among the most common and difficult to control in medical facilities. Pneumonia is also one of the big killers. Should it be the patient's responsibility to see that the floors are properly cleaned in a timely manner? The bacteria thrive in areas where body fluids have accidentally spilled, or where it is wet. If you or your loved one is being maintained in this type of environment, you should bring it to the caregiver's attention and ensure that the room is properly cleaned and sanitized! The risk of infection is too great to allow this type of condition to persist.

Recommending scans, tests, and surgeries that were not needed often place the patient in harms way

With more than five thousand individuals interviewed over the past five years, and experiences within my own family, It was learned that many individuals are having to endure repeated scans or other testing. Why should this be?

One patient underwent intestinal scans to discover the location and source of stomach bleeding caused by medications taken for arthritic pain. Following the first scan, the physician, in reviewing the information, advised that the stomach and intestines had not been adequately emptied and another scan would be required. To the patient's surprise, the same comments were made after the second, third, and fourth scans. Though a fifth scan was recommended, the physician offered no objections when the patient decided there would be no fifth scan.

Would it not be more appropriate after the first scan, to ensure the patient understands the procedures for preparation, or perhaps the physician could hospitalize the patient to ensure proper preparation? Could it be he simply enjoyed the money from all of these scans? In this particular case, stool samples had revealed there was internal bleeding, so why did the physician appear to have more interest in performing scans than finding a way for getting to the root of the problem?

Recently one of the major hospital chains was required to sell a large number of their facilities. This was due to the number of unnecessary heart by-pass surgeries that were performed. How many people want to be put in harm's way to bolster the profits of physicians in this manner? There are frequent reports in the news media of such organizations or medical practitioners being convicted for such crimes. This has not only caused medical costs to go thru the roof, more importantly, the patient is not getting the real care needed. The professionals appear to have no concern or realization of how difficult and painful it is for the ill and/or elderly individuals to undergo these needless tests and surgeries. It is unconscionable that they be made to do so for what appears to be nothing more than a desire for greater profits.

How have these recommendations impacted upon your health?

Many of those interviewed have been negatively affected by the side effects from the various drugs prescribed. Medications taken to lower their cholesterol were alleged to have caused damage to other parts of the body. This included liver and kidney damage, and some reported heart damage from the same drugs that were given to protect the heart! Almost everyone is overly concerned with cholesterol, fat, animal fat, and are fearful to consume beef, pork, milk or eggs due to their fat and cholesterol content

Dr. Ravnskov and Dr. Enig, et al. have clearly dispelled the myths regarding the fat/cholesterol dangers to health. in their critical reviews of the literature.(38), (22) Their conclusions have been confirmed by the many independent scientists who have spoken out in the group called the "The International Network of Cholesterol. Skeptics" (THINCS). (42)

The purpose of this book is to accept their findings, and go beyond their concerns to a new area that appears to have been totally ignored by the health professionals.

I am talking about the connective tissues that make up the support structure of the body. These proteins make up twenty-five percent (25%) of the proteins found in the body! These tissues are virtually omnipresent. They are found in the skin, as the base matrix for bone formation, and surround the various organs, such as the heart and prostate, to prevent enlargement. They provide the elasticity and tensile strength of the circulatory system (arteries), the digestive system, and the pulmonary system. They also give strength and support to the muscles and provide the insulation and strength of the myelin sheath in order to permit normal nerve impulses to be successfully transmitted. They are in every cell of the body including the red blood cells.

The connective tissues are basically multiple strands of protein composed primarily of proline and lysine (amino acids) which are most abundant in animal tissues. They gain their resistance to chemical or physical damage by the process of hydroxylation. Various types of chemical bonds contribute to high tensile strength of these fibers which are, stronger than steel. They also provide the elasticity which allows the lungs, digestive system, heart, arteries, etc. to expand and contract as needed by the body.

Interestingly enough, the connective tissue strands are compressed and wound into very tough bundles of fibers much like a rope or steel cable. If the nutrients needed for repair are not available in the diet as the fibers wear out, deterioration will occur.

Under a microscope the broken fibrils appear as a roughened surface, or something like hangnails. As with any rope, cable, or fabric, the weak spot will only get worse with time due to abrasion or wear. Should this occur on the outside of an artery, this growing weakness could result in the artery ballooning out. This would be diagnosed as an aneurysm. On the other hand, if this weakness were on the inside of the artery, it is very likely that the "hangnails" could eventually result in the formation of a plaque at the site of weakness and ultimately, blockage of the artery.

There seems to be controversy as to what the material is that is removed from blocked arteries. Some reporting it to be cholesterol, some claim white cells, others say platelets. In my opinion it could be anything being transported through the circulatory system to ensure a proper distribution of oxygen, or other nutrients essential to sustain life. Certainly if you reduce the dietary intake of cholesterol by fifty percent you would slow the rate of blockage due to ingested cholesterol.

If one then, through medication with the use of statin drugs, blocks the body's ability to produce cholesterol, then that too would reduce the rate of blockage due to cholesterol simply because there is less of it. This is not necessarily a good thing! This would not have any effect on blockage caused by any other substances.

What appears more important to me is the fact that the body needs cholesterol in every cell if it is to be properly maintained. It has been determined that cholesterol represents 20% of the fat found in the body, much of which is found in the brain and the rest of the nervous system. Failure in the proper transmission of nerve impulses can, and does affect one's ability to think coherently, or to retain control of the muscles for mobility, etc.

Chapter 3

Nutrition — A Brief History

The science of life and the source of good health

This summary on the history of nutrition will look at the first half of the twentieth century compared to the second half. Critical to the building of a good data base for understanding body chemistry and the contributions made by the foods we eat, was the gradual evolution of the analytical tools for identifying those factors that we now know to be the vitamins and trace minerals essential for good health..

In the late 1800s it was found that limes could prevent or reduce the incidence of scurvy on ships. It was not until 1932 that the factor responsible, vitamin C, was isolated. My research seems to confirm that this was indeed the first vitamin to be isolated. Most of the other vitamins were identified and isolated by the late 1950s. This led to the development of dietary rations and/or supplements for the major species of animals including man, the domestic farm animals, and domestic pets. The first vitamin supplements for man became commercially available in the early 1940s.

In the development of our understanding of nutrition and the role it plays in achieving good health., most of the studies were first conducted with small animals, then domestic farm animals and then humans. All of the animals used have numerous similarities with humans.

We share the same basic chemical requirements which enable body functions to be carried out. The basic differences are in the amount of each vitamin, mineral, amino acids, fatty acids, etc., which are more directly related to the size of the animal rather than the species.

Structurally the species mentioned above are very similar:

- They have bone support structures
- They have hepatic Systems (livers)
- They have circulatory systems (arteries and veins)
- They have digestive systems (cattle and sheep have more stomachs and eat forage crops with an ability to end up with the same basic chemicals as the animals that have single stomachs.)
- They have pulmonary systems that include lungs
- They have spleens
- They have hearts (though not all have four chambers as humans do.)
- They have nervous systems. (Despite the differences in complexity, the nature of the transmission of nerve impulses is not all that different between the species.)
- They have an outer skin, the composition of which is very similar for all species. (Some animals, such as dogs, do not

perspire through the skin, but maintain fluid loss through their tongue.

It was through the rations and supplements available at that time that farmers were able to overcome many of their animals' health problems which were caused by malnutrition. This resulted in healthier offspring, better rate of growth and greater profitability in the production of cattle, swine, poultry, and other farm animals.

It was not until the late 1950s that the recommendations for humans were changed dramatically. Instead of recommending a daily vitamin based on the Recommended Daily Allowance (RDA), the HOD promoted the concept, via the USDA, that it is better for us to get all of our nutrition from the foods we consume, based upon the food pyramids and the food guidelines. We were then discouraged from taking a daily supplement!

Science has learned much over the centuries about the composition of animals and the role that nutrition plays in the health of all animals, including humans. The most significant difference between the domestic animals and humans is that of **choice.** The farm animals as well as domestic pets are fed what their owners want them to have, while humans have a choice as to what they eat. Many individuals would like to eat a healthy diet in order to be healthy. However, this is no easy task. The different recommendations that have been put fourth by the HOD have been observed to change frequently for reasons unknown. Almost daily one can hear or read reports that are in conflict. How can a person know who or what to believe — what is or is not good for one's health?

Nutrition as we know it today represents the very basis for a healthy life. Without the complete and balanced diet, good baseline nutrition cannot be established or maintained. It is much like building a home, where the basic foundation must be sound and on bedrock as well as having reinforcement, if it is to survive the storms of time.

I know of no science that is more critical to achieving good health than the application of nutrition for the prevention and cure of chronic diseases. It is with amazement that I see the HOD virtually denying the very existence of nutrition in their pursuit of providing medical services to their patients. Of course, the practice of medicine would be far less profitable should the physician include basic nutritional concepts in his or her practice.

This would take them from making people well, to making people healthy! That is not the business of medicine, as viewed by the HOD.

Chapter 4

The Great Deception — Human versus Animal Nutrition

What are the real differences in nutritional needs?

So why do you feed your dog a good diet, and choose a poor diet for yourself? Is it the recommendations of the government, your personal trainer, your health food clerk, your physician? Or is it the recommendations of the American Heart Association, or the USDA? Or do you just believe in the food pyramids and the food guidelines?

There are a great number of independent scientists, not a part of the HOD that tend to agree with me, that the new guidelines and the old ones, the new food pyramids, and the old ones, do not represent what would be in your best interest, for achieving good health..

The concern expressed by those in the medical profession, when I make the comparison of human nutrition to that of the farm animals and domestic pets is usually alarm. They have advised that the two cannot be compared because of all the differences. When asked to describe some of the differences, they talk about the different enzymes between the species and other compounds produced by the body. My basic point is that it is not the chemical compounds that each species must produce, but rather, what are the chemicals required for each species to produce these various compounds. The basic chemicals are extremely similar even though each species may be programmed through genetics to make slightly different species-specific end products from these chemicals.

I think this can be better understood if we take practical common sense into the equation of life. The current understanding of nutrition is based primarily on the early work with many other animals prior to confirming these truths on humans. Prior to 1960 the general teachings were that similarities out numbered differences between the species. This was true for almost every chemical evaluated for its nutritional contribution, and that chemical's function in each of the different species.

Strangely enough, the USDA supported the development of animal feeds, pet foods, and human foods to improve the nutritional status of all species. In about 1960, their support of animal nutrition continued and continues to this day with great success. The farm animals are healthy and profitable and *to a lesser degree*, the domestic pets are quite healthy due to their continued support and the use of RDA based diets.

With my emphasis on meat, milk, and eggs as the best way to prevent chronic diseases among humans, one individual raised a very legitimate question. Do the domestic animals eat these foods? The simple answer is yes. Their mothers, except for chickens and turkeys nurse their off spring. Baby animals are frequently fed cow's milk or milk products such as slopping the hogs with whey from milk or the dried material may be incorporated in their rations. Meat and bone meal is a common ingredient in their rations.

Recent reports of an increasing incidence of cancer in dogs over the past 10-20 years came as no surprise to me. When considering the changes that have taken place in the manufacture of pet foods in recent years, it tends to confirm my theories that nutrition is directly related to the incidence of some cancers.

Changes in the regulatory standards for the manufacture of pet foods are believed to be causal for the reported increase in cancer among dogs. This could apply to other species as well. The major changes observed would be expected to take the nutritional safety margin away that had been built into their complete and balanced formulations. I feel confident these products meet the testing required for their nutritional claims—just that the safety net is gone, should the animals be stressed or exposed to infections.

These changes were more likely dictated by market forces than anything else because:

1. The decline in beef and pork production with the concurrent increase in chicken and turkey production. This reduces the use of meat by-products while increasing poultry by-product use. (I consider meat by-products the better food for pets)
2. The HOD recommendations for humans to avoid foods containing cholesterol virtually eliminated the use of beef, pork, milk products or eggs from these formulations. This I believe was more a fear by the marketing moguls that pet owners were going to reject their

products when reading the labels and finding these foods included.

Comparison of Regulatory Standards*

Adult Dog Food	1975	Current
Moisture, Maximum	78%	82%
Protein, Minimum	12%	8%
Fat, Minimum	6%	3%

*Ash and Crude Fiber Standards remain unchanged

What would you expect when reducing the protein by 33%, the fat by 50% and adding 4% more water? There is no question but that the nutritional value would be compromised, and yes, I would expect under stress, chronic diseases could become a problem. Perhaps this can be better understood using the following theoretical reformulation:

Composition of 20 pounds of meat or poultry by-products:

Component	%	Contains
Moisture	72%	14.4 pounds
Protein	20%	4.0 pounds
Fat	15%	3.0 pounds

> If one simply removes 20 pounds of meat by-products from 100 pounds of formula, replacing it with 19.5 pounds of water plus 0.5 pounds of vegetable gum to gel the product by binding the water, the product would require the same ingredient statement and would meet the new guaranteed analysis for moisture, protein, and fat. Thus 20 pounds of meat by-products are replaced with 19.5 pounds of water plus 0.5 pounds of carbohydrate! The remaining meat by-products in the formulation would be replaced with poultry by-products. Do you think this would marginalize the nutritional value of the product? This appears to be what has happened!
>
> Unfortunately, these types of changes occur frequently in human foods as well, adversely affecting the nutritional status of humans. I will address the need to better understand food labels in Book III of this series.

For reasons unknown, around 1960 the USDA position on human nutrition and health took a significant turn. The earlier recommendations were generally reversed. Animal fat, cholesterol, cholesterol containing foods, vitamin and mineral supplements, beef, pork, milk and eggs were no longer considered good foods. In their stead, they recommended chicken, turkey, soy products, and the food pyramids and food guidelines.

What is hard to understand, is the fact that the farm animals were relatively free of chronic diseases in the 1950s and that continues to this day. Humans on the other hand, with the support of the USDA and others in the HOD, have experienced nothing but increasing chronic diseases. This has come as a result of their specific recommendations for humans that differ so much from their recommendations for the farm animals that continue to be healthy and profitable. What do you think is responsible for this change? It cannot be that the nutritional needs for humans have changed!

There are numerous suggestions offered for the lack of chronic diseases among the farm animals — such as: They don't live as long as humans: they have different genetics; they have different nutritional needs;

The truth of the matter is that:

- Animals deprived of good nutrition do have chronic diseases, similar to humans.
- The breeding herds and flocks have long lives for their species.
- Most of the farm animals are fed commercially prepared feeds to ensure good health. and profitability.
- The genetic pool of the farm animals and domestic pets is probably no better or worse than with humans.
- Humans have CHOICE in their diets as the major difference from the farm animals and domestic pets.

- The recommendations for sustaining good health among humans, pets, and farm animals should be based upon RDA type diets including appropriate supplements for the individual species and life cycle.

In my opinion the recommendations of the HOD have critically compromised the basic foundation of the human body. The primary support structure of the body has been put in jeopardy in those individuals who would care, or dare, to follow their recommendations. Why can't people be allowed, and taught to eat foods that will make them healthy?

The Chemicals Needed for Complete and Balanced Nutrition of Humans and the Domestic Animals

With humans, the chemicals found in foods do not make for a complete and balanced diet as evidenced by the prevalence of chronic diseases. The basic chemicals needed by the various species are essentially the same. It is true that some animals have the ability to produce some vitamins , amino acids, fats, etc. that other animals cannot produce. This does not represent a significant difference between the species as to what is required for good health, but rather, how will these chemical be provided. Will those chemicals be present in the foods consumed or provided in supplemental rations or through vitamin and mineral supplements?

The following chemicals are necessary for any animal to sustain good baseline nutrition. The amount of each chemical will depend upon the species, age, gender, size, and stage of life. Many of these chemicals have recommended usage levels, while others are known to be needed, but no recommended levels have been established.

Vitamins

Biotin	Vitamin B_1	Vitamin D
Folic Acid	Vitamin B_2	Vitamin E
Niacin	Vitamin B_6	Vitamin K
Pantothenic Acid	Vitamin B_{12}	
Vitamin A	Vitamin C	

Minerals

Calcium	Molybdenum
Chloride	Nickel
Chromium	Phosphorus
Cobalt	Potassium
Copper	Selenium
Fluorine	Silicon
Iodine	Sodium
Iron	Sulfur
Magnesium	Vanadium
Manganese	Zinc

Amino Acids

Alanine	Tryptophan*
Serine	Proline
Threonine*	Hydroxyproline
Valine*	Aspartic Acid
Leucine*	Glutamic Acid
Isolucine*	Histidine*
Phenylalanine*	Arginine*
Tyrosine	Lysine*
Cysteine	Hydroxylysine
Cystine	Taurine
Methonine*	

* Essential in diet, most animals cannot produce.

Fats (Unsaturated Fatty Acids)

Oleic
Linoleic
Linolenic
Arachidonic

Carbohydrates are not as critical to good health as the vitamins, minerals, amino acids, and fats, except that an excess plays a role in obesity and other chronic diseases.

Water is certainly the most critical to support good health, but like the other chemicals, one can have too little or too much.

Chapter 5

Why the HOD approach to prevention of chronic diseases is not working

Does the HOD have a hidden agenda that has nothing to do with disease prevention?

There have been two recent reports of using MRI evaluations to diagnose early onset of Alzheimer's disease and bipolar disorder, by identifying deterioration of the myelin sheath that insulates the nerves. What I can't figure out is, is this technique designed to sell MRI scans, or is it to prevent or cure? They reported treatments are available to rid the patient of free radicals via vitamins C and E. There was no mention in the reports suggesting repair of the myelin sheaths through dietary change!

I cannot over emphasize the role that I believe the trace minerals have in achieving good health.. I see it as an absolute necessity that people take a good vitamin-mineral supplement, based on the RDAs. I think it's equally mandatory that we initiate a program that'll help us to identify truly, in honesty, if there are other factors that should be incorporated into the RDAs; not what I consider their lame attempts to degrade the better RDAs that were established in '68 and '80.

If one takes a look at the number of people affected by one or more of the chronic diseases over the past half century, there is no room for doubt that we have more diseases. It is equally true that more and more of the population is being affected by these diseases. Many people experience multiple forms of chronic diseases.

The question that I would like to have answered is this — how come things are getting worse after fifty years of their recommendations? We have been told these recommendations were the way to a more healthful life.

One cannot say the cause is that many have not followed their advice. The evidence is clear from food consumption patterns that their recommendations have had an enormous effect on production and consumption of food.

The consumption of eggs per person in 1945 was 420 – 425 per year. In 2000 the per capita consumption was below 250 per year. This is less than sixty percent (60%) of what it was in 1945. The beef, pork, and dairy industries were devastated by their recommendations. This gave rise to very significant increases in the chicken, turkey and soy protein industries.

If these recommendations were of any value, why aren't more people healthy? These recommendations were designed to make people very unhealthy, giving rise to increasing the incidence of chronic diseases.

What is the evidence for this belief?

They:

- Only treat the symptom, never the cause
- Seek only the cure, never the cause
- Recommend dietary policies designed to cause chronic diseases

- Never consider RDA type nutritional supplements as a treatment to prevent or cure chronic diseases
- Speak with "one voice"
- Are quick to blame genetics as the probable cause, when they don't know the answer
- Say chronic diseases have no known cause, are incurable and require lifetime medications or surgeries.
- Use fear tactics — predict coronaries, strokes, blocked arteries, require amputations, or other surgeries, etc.
- Prescribe medications that they know may cause addiction, damage organs such as kidneys, liver, bones, muscles, etc., that result in more chronic diseases. This is known as "collateral damage."
- Never advise the low risk and low cost of improving your health by taking an RDA based multiple vitamin/mineral supplements.
- Every mistake a health professional makes appears to enhance their profits; however, those mistakes not only cost you more, but often increase your risk of pain or even death.

Searching for Cures

Let us look at cause and prevention of diseases as is practiced in the medical field today. Before we had so many chronic diseases, the HOD spent most of their research seeking the cause of the infectious diseases. They found that bacteria and viruses were the primary causes for diseases such as polio, typhoid, pneumonia, malaria, tetanus, diphtheria, measles, mumps, bubonic plague, smallpox and numerous other infectious diseases. They learned better sanitation practices to reduce the spread of the diseases, but it took the development of vaccines and antibiotics to prevent such diseases as polio, smallpox and many others.

Infectious diseases such as polio or small pox are known to kill or cripple, and the search for prevention, as well as some cures, has proven successful with the development of vaccines for each disease. Treatment for the diseases, once contracted, in some cases prevented death, but often left the patient with severe disabilities and major scarring. Use of vaccines has been exceedingly effective in disease prevention.

The tactics used in the medical professions for control of non-infectious, chronic diseases, has been totally different. The basic approach appears to be to **ignore the cause** and **find the cure.** In the meantime, diagnose, treat and provide care with little interest devoted to research efforts aimed at identifying the cause of the various chronic diseases, so that prevention would be the order of the day. To prevent or cure the chronic diseases would be counter to the business interest of the medical professionals.

One good example of this would be Arthritis. There are more than one hundred (100) forms of this disease, and in general terms, this is not a killer disease. It is generally believed to result from degeneration of the cartilage, collagen, and/or elastin found between the joints in the body. Extensive research effort has been expended over the years to develop pain medications that temporarily relieve the pain. Over time, the body appears to find a way to get around such pain blockers in order to signal a problem that needs to be fixed.

One hundred million dollars was the reported cost for the development of one pain medication, and one billion for the next generation pain medicine. This information was presented in TV advertisements by two of the major pharmaceutical companies in recent years.

The development of artificial joints and their implantation over recent years has met with considerable success. Only limited research effort has been directed toward identifying the cause of the degeneration of these tissues or the body's lack of ability to replace or repair these tissues. In my opinion, the solution to this problem would be quite inexpensive and would negate the need for many of the pain medications and the various joint replacement surgeries taking place in our country today.

Not too long ago I was watching a news cast on TV that dealt with Parkinson's disease. A guest celebrity was being interviewed. If I heard him correctly, he said that he was not at all interested in what may have caused him to contract the disease, but rather was only concerned with finding a cure! A recent Telethon for muscular dystrophy was asking financial supporters to help them **find a**

cure. They have been searching for the cure for at least thirty years! There are many fund raisers to raise money to search for the cure for cancer, multiple sclerosis, and indeed, for most of the chronic diseases. The money raised and spent over the past half century has to be in the billions of dollars.

I have found No examples of research projects being funded that were designed to find the cause of any of the chronic diseases. One organization, the Alzheimer's Foundation allocated five percent (5%) of their funded projects for diet and health. studies.(2) That is 5% of 183 million dollars, — less than 10 million dollars over a twenty year period. Bear in mind that diet and health studies may or may not be concerned with finding the cause.

In conducting my review of these various organizations, I was amazed to learn of the funds that have been raised over the past fifty years in search of cures for the various diseases. I am not advocating that such funding be stopped.
I *do* urge the philanthropic groups or individuals funding the research. for these organizations, to review their annual reports, to see what research grants are being funded, and insist that some portion of their monies fund research that would help find the cause of the diseases. When the cause is known, it is much easier to identify appropriate measures to prevent — or possibly cure the disease in question.
And what if it were as easy as changing their diets?

To advise a person to consume foods that would support the maintenance and repair of the collagen, elastin, and cartilage would, if effective, eliminate the need for a lot of pain medications and joint replacement surgeries. However, this would adversely affect the income and profits of the HOD.

On the other hand, if their recommendations were to cause one <u>to avoid</u> the foods that could provide these important chemicals, essential to the replacement and repair of these connective tissues, then it is reasonable to expect to see an increased need for the pain medications and surgeries.. This, in turn would ensure that their desire for more business and profits would be achieved!

In my opinion, this is exactly what they have done with the simple recommendations that people avoid animal fats and cholesterol. This precludes the consumption of beef, pork, milk and eggs which are the primary sources of the chemicals needed to build and maintain these connective tissues. These chemicals are common, primarily in some animal tissues!

<u>Note</u>: Unpublished research on the connective tissues of various species of animals, including chicken, turkey, pork, and beef, clearly show that the larger the animal, the more abundant the connective tissues, and the higher the tensile strength. The poultry meats, chicken and turkey, contain the smallest amount of connective tissues and were much weaker as a support structure. This was consistent with the actual needs of the animals. As the size and weight of the animal increases, the organs are larger and require bigger bones, lungs,

digestive systems, etc., thus requiring the connective tissues to be more abundant and considerably stronger. Pigs are closest to the size, (in weight) of humans, and this may be why pig hearts have been considered for possible implant in humans. The stents used for replacing defective arteries in humans are made from a fraction of collagen found in pigs.

Numerous other diseases are attributable to deterioration of connective tissues:

The Circulatory System Diseases

- The external surface of the arteries become less pliable as the fat content (fat, fatty acids and cholesterol) is reduced. This causes the arteries to become more brittle, and contributes to **Hardening of The Arteries**.
- The gradual deterioration of the collagen causes the arteries to lose tensile strength and elasticity when the diet does not provide adequate nutrients for the formation and/or repair of these tissues. Variations in blood pressure can cause formation of a balloon effect in the weakened section of an artery. This is called an **Aneurysm.** Should this balloon burst, there is a hemorrhage, and the loss of blood can be fatal if not treated immediately.
- The internal surface of the artery (lumen) is dependent upon various chemicals such as fat, for lubricity and pliability, intact

collagen, and elastin to provide tensile strength, elasticity and a very smooth surface. This expedites the flow of blood and nutrients being transported throughout the body, including the most distal parts such as the toes, fingers and of course, the brain. It is my opinion, that as the strands of collagen or elastin fragment, that the ends of the broken fibers act much like a "hang nail", causing the snagging of large chemical compounds such as cholesterol, fibrin, white cells, platelets, or any other components contained in the blood as it flows past the damaged area of the arterial inner wall. Over time this could cause a **Blockage of the Artery**. The literature suggests there are several thoughts regarding the chemical constituents found at the site of blockages. Some contend that the material is nothing more than cholesterol, while others believe that it is nothing but white cells.

The reason for these various opinions could be that it is not any one material — just whatever happens to get snagged. The chemical analysis is simple enough, so why has this difference of opinion not been conclusively resolved over the past fifty years? I would go a step beyond and suggest that the following scenario could be quite possible:

The HOD contends that cholesterol is the cause for blocked arteries, as well as the material to be found in the blockages. If true, this would support the need to lower cholesterol. Statin drugs like Lipitor and Zocor are used to lower cholesterol. They act by blocking the body's production of cholesterol and CO Q10, a co-enzyme essential for proper metabolism. Common sense says that if you reduce the number of molecules of cholesterol by restricting dietary intake by fifty percent (50%), and blocking the production by the body, this would, of necessity, reduce the number of molecules that could be snagged by at least fifty percent (50%)!

The problem that I see with this approach is that:

1. The body needs cholesterol. It is present in every cell of the body and is believed to play a role in the cell wall support structure. Along with collagen and elastin, cholesterol must be present if the cells are to withstand the pressures of doing their job.

2. The body produces cholesterol based upon need. If there is ample in the body, it produces less, and if there is not enough, it will produce more. This happens regardless of dietary cholesterol intake. This has been well established.

3. If the production of cholesterol is blocked with chemicals used to lower the cholesterol in the plasma, I believe it becomes a "shipping" problem. Department A is calling the factory asking for more

cholesterol, and the factory is unable to ship the amount needed for proper body function.

What is the likely net effect from this shortage? There are many possibilities, but the one that scares me the most is that structures such as the myelin sheath which provides the insulation for the individual nerves, could act like spark plug wires on a car that have no insulation. There would be some "shorting out" which could best be described as neurological diseases such as bipolar disorder, schizophrenia, Parkinson's and perhaps all of the non-infectious, neurological diseases. The myelin sheath contains collagen and elastin for tensile strength and elasticity, in addition to its function of keeping the electrical nerve impulses isolated, to ensure the transmission of the signal is completed. It stands to reason that proper function is dependent on these chemicals, including cholesterol, if one is to have an intact myelin sheath protecting each nerve.

The Communicable Disease Prevention Center (CDC) has reported that of the total medical costs in the U.S., approximately:

> **Twenty five percent (25%)** are for the treatment of infectious diseases (HIV, aids, measles, mumps, polio, typhoid fever, limes disease, small pox, chicken pox, diphtheria, pneumonia, etc.), industrial accidents, in-home accidents, traffic accidents, gun shot wounds, domestic violence, and various causes such as

accidental chemical poisoning, microbiological toxins such as Botulinum, Salmonella, Staphylococcal, etc.

Seventy five percent (75%) are for the treatment of chronic diseases that include, but are not limited to, such diseases as arthritis (more than one hundred different types), strokes, heart attacks (CHD), hardening of the arteries (arteriosclerosis), COPD (bronchitis and emphysema), hypertension, aneurisms, dementia, Alzheimer's disease, type II diabetes, obesity, psoriasis, gout, autism, bi-polar disorder, schizophrenia, numerous forms of cancer involving the skin and any or all of the organs within the body. This category of diseases is estimated to be ninety percent (90%), due to nutritional deficiencies! They are not caused by bacteria, yeasts, molds, viruses, fungi, and **only rarely** can they be positively connected to genetics as the causal factor. Another way of describing the chronic diseases is to say they are the "man made" diseases. This is due primarily to the flawed recommendations of the HOD, or the neglect of individuals in taking proper care of their nutritional needs, due to either a lack of knowledge or a lack of concern.

Searching in All The Wrong Places?

Over the past five years I have reviewed hundreds, if not thousands, of the organizations operating in the areas of health and medicine. Some of the more well known included:

- The United States Department of Agriculture (USDA)
- The National Institutes of Health (NIH)
- The National Academy of Sciences (NAS)
- The National Research Council (NRC)
- The Communicable Disease Prevention Center (CDC)
- The U.S. Food and Drug Administration (FDA)
- The American Heart Association (AHA)
- The American Cancer Society (ACS)
- The American Diabetic Association (ADA)
- The American Association of Dietetics
- The Muscular Dystrophy Foundation
- The Multiple Sclerosis Foundation
- The Mayo Clinic
- Johns-Hopkins University

The objective for searching the literature was to learn what is being said, compared to what is being done regarding:

- What their mission statements revealed.
- To discern their position on the cause, prevention, or cure for chronic diseases.

- The type(s) of research. projects funded
- The sources of monies for research.

The results were expected to shine some light on why, over the past half century, we experienced such an enormous increase in non-infectious, chronic diseases in the U.S. What I learned was that in almost every instance, it is very important to read between the lines, to see what is not being said or done!

Almost universally, they speak of prevention along with the numerous flawed "one voice" recommendations cited earlier. The problem that I see with their use of the word prevention is that it is but a false veil, leading people to believe they truly are concerned with disease prevention. I found a review of the CDC web page and searchable records to be quite interesting. This is equally true of most other medical sites and those of the various foundations who purport to have a keen interest in ridding the world of a particular disease. With the CDC, it is interesting that numerous programs have been developed, under the guise of promoting disease prevention through community programs across the country. These programs, costing millions of dollars each year, are basically awareness programs to promote the recommendations of the HOD. If one were truly interested in disease prevention, it seems plausible that some of those monies would be better spent on determining the cause of the disease in question. Do they really believe that simply telling people of the risk factors for diseases, (mostly erroneous) along with their recommendations will ***prevent*** that disease?

I believe that you prevent the disease when *you know the cause,* and then take the necessary steps to correct whatever has been causal in the first place. This would be far more effective than any *awareness program*, especially when they acknowledge that the cause remains unknown! This makes about as much sense as telling someone the way to prevent polio is to not go near anyone who has it! This is ***avoidance*** of the disease rather than ***prevention***. It may keep some from getting it, but does this really prevent polio? It took the development of a vaccine to prevent such an infectious disease.

If we consider arthritis, which is believed by many, to be caused by deterioration of the tissues supporting the bone joints, would it not make more sense to determine what causes the deterioration? Then the HOD could provide the information that would allow a person to prevent deterioration. From the patient's point of view, this would be much more effective (less painful, less expensive, and less debilitating) than for the HOD to find ways to slow the progression of the disease with lifetime medication or surgery, as is the common practice.

This is the consistent pattern I observed in reviewing virtually every organization, be it public or private, when it comes to the search for cures of the various non-infectious, chronic diseases. Enough of this is enough! Let us use the public funds and the donations to find the truth, and prevent and possibly cure these many diseases — NOW!

To further your understanding of what I am writing, included here are reviews of only two of the numerous organizations that I have researched. This is not intended to "pick on" any particular organization, but merely examples of my observations. I believe they typify what I have observed with virtually every organization I have reviewed. The longer I search, the greater the confirmation of my belief that the majority of research being funded with billions of dollars over the past fifty years is intentionally directed toward finding a treatment, (medication or surgery) rather than toward a prevention or cure..

I should advise you that due to the substantial amount of monies being donated in search of cures for the various chronic diseases, there has arisen numerous look-alike or sound-alike organizations that take away many of the donations. Individuals think they are supporting one organization, but are, in fact, donating to a look alike.

One of the organizations I reviewed was the National Multiple Sclerosis Society. "The List of Current Research Projects Funded in 2005" has some very interesting research projects. Again, this review is intended as an example only, and is not intended to single out one particular organization. The concerns that I identify with the MS Society are the same with other organizations that I have reviewed, and as I said, there have been hundreds.

In the listing for the fall of 2005, there were three hundred and nineteen grants awarded, with some covering one to five years. The grants ranged from $11,407.00 to $4.8 million. They are listed by state and country, but most are in the U.S. The fifteen various categories of research projects include:

- Human Genetics
- Measuring MS disease activity
- Immunology
- Epidemiology
- Rehabilitation
- Neurophysiology
- CNS repair
- Biology of Glia
- Infectious agents
- Psychosocial aspects of MS
- Tissue/DNA Banks
- Biochemistry/Biophysics.
- Health Care Delivery/Policy
- Diagnostic Methods
- Therapy/Management of MS

"The mission of the National Multiple Sclerosis Society is to end the devastating effects of MS."

From the lay man's point of view, it appears that the largest grant of 4.8 million dollars is designed to find better methods of detecting damaged nerve fibers (diagnostics), and agents (medications) that would prevent the nervous system from further damage.

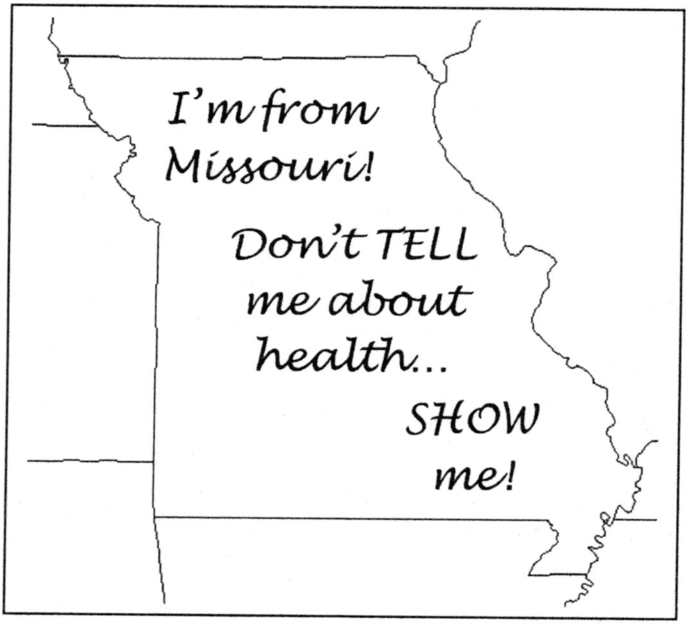
I'm from
Missouri!
Don't TELL
me about
health...
SHOW
me!

And **being** from Missouri — using my "red neck logic," — I suggest the following scenario might be worth considering as a less expensive and faster way to learn the cause, and perhaps the prevention and/or cure of MS.

- When we come into this world, most babies get here quite healthy provided the parents were reasonably healthy.
- The body is programmed to repair itself through genetics, if properly nourished.

- From birth, I believe it is a given, that all cells of whatever type will eventually deteriorate and automatically be replaced if the person (or other animal) is well nourished. It has been claimed that the total cells in the body are replaced about every seven years.
- The old question of "which came first, the chicken or the egg?" might well be asked as "which came first, nutrition or genes?" I believe nutrition came first! Genes don't make nutrients, but genes use nutrients to make whatever material they are programmed to manufacture. I believe that it takes good baseline nutrition to have good genes. Domestic animals appear to have good genes due to the low incidence of chronic diseases in those animals. It is certain that most domestic animals receive complete and balanced diets, while it is equally certain humans do not!
- Of the 319 research. projects being funded, there is not one word mentioned about nutritional research and how it relates to the cause of MS. Why?

My concern is that even if they did pursue nutrition research based upon the current philosophy for healthy eating, they would still not find the cause. Remember, for thirty years, beef pork, milk, eggs, and multi vitamin and mineral supplements were for the most part forbidden, and now are seriously restricted in their recommendations. With domestic animals, there are no forbidden foods! Of course there are a number of poisonous plants that can harm man and animals alike.

Risk Factors for Diseases

We are constantly reminded of the risk of having a stroke, heart attack, hardening of the arteries, type II diabetes, obesity, and the list goes on, one scare tactic after another. We are to avoid smoking, animal fats, cholesterol, numerous foods, etc. etc.

There is little doubt that the greatest of the risk factors facing mankind is the lack of achieving a *complete and balanced diet*. This is the *only* path to what I call *good baseline nutrition*. This is, without question, the major cause for the non-infectious, chronic diseases that are being experienced by the human population.

I think we should be aware of risk factors that could cause medical problems; but I think we should consider all known factors, many of which are never mentioned by medical professionals. There is no doubt that some things represent a much higher risk than others, and the *relative level of risk* should be considered. Virtually everything represents a risk, dependent on amount and frequency. There may be a lower limit below which one should not go, and likewise, there is usually an upper limit that could cause harm. Too much of a good thing is not good, just as, not enough of a good thing is cause for concern This is especially true if it has to do with the vitamins, minerals, trace minerals, amino acids, fatty acids, fiber, proteins, carbohydrates, and other factors essential for good baseline nutrition.

It is a serious problem when the risks for disease are not based upon all the facts. To tell a patient they are at risk for a disease when there is only junk science to support the claimed risk, is deception of the worst kind! This is the case with the claims that animal fats and cholesterol will cause one to have clogged arteries, heart attacks, and strokes. There are no legitimate scientific studies to support these claims.

There are major risks associated with many of the medications being prescribed each and every day by those in the HOD. The medications frequently are used for treating only the symptom, while the side effects have been known to cause the patient to experience such problems as kidney failure, liver damage, suicidal tendencies, muscle deterioration, or even coronary heart disease. These side effects are often provided in very fine print, filling an entire page in some of the journals in which the products are being advertised. These disclosures are required by law, but with such fine print, I doubt that many patients take the time to read them. By default, they find at a later time — perhaps too late — that the new problems they are experiencing are side effects from their medications. We hear of this too often, as products are being withdrawn from the markets.

I would argue that the recommendations of the HOD, based upon their risk factors, are designed to create chronic diseases, rather than

reduce the incidence of chronic diseases. So much better for their business!

Risk factor enumeration has proven to be an effective fear tactic. We see it being used every day in TV advertisements, on the radio, in newspapers and magazines, on the internet, and other media sources. They strive to sell all manner of scans or tests, as well as new surgeries like gastric bypass for obesity. Some of these procedures carry considerable risk, but they are down played until it is too late!

If we take alcohol as an example, it is reasonable to consider the risk. I do not concur that an all or none attitude gives proper clarity to assess the true risk. Bear in mind, with an addict it should be all or none, but I am talking of the non-addict. The adverse health effect will surely be there if one drinks a fifth a day. But what about the person who has a glass of wine each day; or a glass each month, or perhaps one glass a year? I think that you would agree that one glass a year will do no harm to the health of a non-addict. Some believe it would help one to be healthier.

It is the frequency and the amount of a substance that determines the health effect. Often, the HOD uses risk factors to create a belief among the populous that it is the all or none concept that should be followed. As with eggs in the late 1950s, their recommendation was to consume no more than one egg per week, and then throw the yolk away. By looking at <u>their data</u> on the composition of foods, it is clear that egg whites contain zero fat and zero cholesterol! So, how sensible is it to have such a limit on eggs if you throw the yolks away? Of course, they have, forty years later, said it was ok to eat one per day, including the yolk! What happened to the risk factor? I know several individuals who to this day practice the earlier recommendation of one egg per week, and many eat none or one a month.

I believe this is the type of fallacious and irresponsible recommendations from the HOD that cause many people to have difficulty in achieving good health.

Perspectives on Chronic Diseases

I view the non-infectious, chronic diseases to be very unique in our population. There are almost daily announcements of a new disorder, syndrome, or disease that has been discovered or diagnosed.

In the developing countries, infectious diseases are the top priority. While there is frequent evidence of malnutrition in many countries, the occurrence of many of the non-infectious, chronic diseases, when compared to the U.S., are not at all common. Could this be because they can't afford to have these types of diseases, due to their lack of money?

I believe they do incur these diseases, but with a much lower incidence. The neurological diseases, such as attention deficit disorder, attention deficit hyperactivity disorder, Alzheimer's disease, dementia, arthritis of various types, blockages of the arteries, aneurisms, irritable bowel syndrome, the various forms of cancer, prostate enlargement, etc., were of low incidence in this country in the 1950s. Indeed, most had not even been created! I consider many of the non-infectious diseases to have been "man-made," caused by the erroneous recommendations that have been forthcoming from the HOD over the last fifty years.

During my youth in the 1930s and 1940s, I can recall the farm animals and humans having various chronic diseases. This was certainly less frequent than can be observed today. There were fewer types of the non-infectious diseases affecting man and animals. In the late 1940s, the diet was more meat, milk, and eggs with fruits and vegetables and grain products; and it was at this time in history, that multi vitamins and minerals were first used to reinforce the diets of all animals, including man. It was not until the late 1950s that the HOD, with their recommendations, started to demonize the good foods and discourage the use of vitamin and mineral supplements for humans. Note: *That has never been the policy or practice with the farm animals or domestic pets.* Since that time, those animals have always received these supplements, and have had ever improving health to this day in the area of non-infectious, chronic diseases. It was last reported that in the U.S., 9.5 billion broilers are raised each year. If you include all of the other animals being raised over the past fifty years, that would be approaching a trillion animals.

What is most interesting is that the incidence of non-infectious, chronic diseases among the animals is almost non-existent. In reviewing this with veterinarians, they estimated about three percent incidence among the farm animals. This tells me, in no uncertain terms, that good nutrition has prevented many of the non-infectious, chronic diseases among the animals! Since nutritional studies were first conducted with the animals, and this knowledge was later confirmed to be just as effective in humans in almost all instances, then it appears logical to believe that these diseases in humans could be prevented in the same manner. The only problem that I find, is that the recommendations, to avoid the good foods, (meat, milk, and eggs), along with discouraging the use of vitamin and mineral supplements for humans, coincides with — and has been causal in — humans experiencing these diseases. The longer this continues, the worse it will become!

The solutions being offered for obesity by the HOD are bariatric treatment or gastric by-pass surgery. Gastric by-pass is reported to be $20 thousand per person. Simpler, safer, and less expensive approaches are available, and this gives cause for serious questions to be raised. Recent estimates show twenty five to fifty percent of the population is either obese or morbidly obese. Only recently has obesity been accepted as a medical condition. Wow, this is going to get expensive, but **who will be paying for it**? Of those whom I have interviewed over recent years who have had gastric by-pass surgery, many have reported having major problems with the surgery. To begin with, it is reported that approximately five percent will die of complications from the surgery within a year. This affects mostly men. Two of the women interviewed advised they had each had the surgery seven years earlier. Each of them had endured six subsequent surgeries to repair problems caused by the surgery, and each continued to have problems with eating disorders. It has been reported elsewhere that some individuals who have the surgery gradually eat more, allowing the stomach to stretch, so that they are back where they were before the surgery. They have proven that this can cause a person to lose weight with the surgery, but it may not be permanent, and it can be very dangerous.

They appear to have found a niche for nutrition after all. The HOD is now contemplating ways to shore up your nutrition by way of genetic manipulation. A recent article from Tuffs University is declaring this to be the way of the future. (46) Not an inexpensive process to be sure! One thing you can be certain of is that we can't afford to do this with every cow, pig or chicken, nor do we need to! I am certain that, unless the individual receiving such genetic modification has good base line nutrition prior to the modification, any benefits from the treatment will be short lived. I suppose their next step in this developmental process will be to have this declared to be a "medical condition" so that Medicare and the health insurance companies will then cover most of the cost. But <u>who</u> will be paying for it?
Please, let's use a little common sense here.

My first recollection of attention deficit disorder being diagnosed is almost classic. I thought this was a new replacement for discipline! After all, it was about this time in our history that political correctness was being implemented.

The old adage of "spare the rod and spoil the child" represented the fear factor most used in parenting, as well as in the educational facilities. I know that it was the fear of discipline that kept me on the straight and narrow, even-though I do not remember ever receiving the discipline most feared. Fear alone did the trick!

When they transferred this fear factor from the children to the parents and school administrators, the children knew they had a green light to do almost anything without fear of discipline. At the same time, parents and school administrators were fearful, and still are, of the legal reprisals possible from children's services or their children, should they dare to administer discipline. Drugs became the new discipline.

This approach to discipline, coupled with their recommendations resulting in malnutrition, shows me that attention deficit disorder is indeed a "man-made" disease, along with many other non-infectious, chronic diseases. The literature reports that deterioration of the myelin sheath is found with several of the neurological diseases. They don't know the cause for the deterioration, but they do have medications that are said to slow the progression of the disease.

Would it not be far more appropriate to determine how to repair it than to attempt to slow the rate of deterioration? As a cut finger will be healed by the body, so can the deterioration of the myelin sheath be stopped and/or repaired — through proper nutrition! But this is never tried or even considered. Could it be the fear of losing a patient (and income) if cured?

Who would dare to kill this Golden Goose? I would dare — with good nutrition!

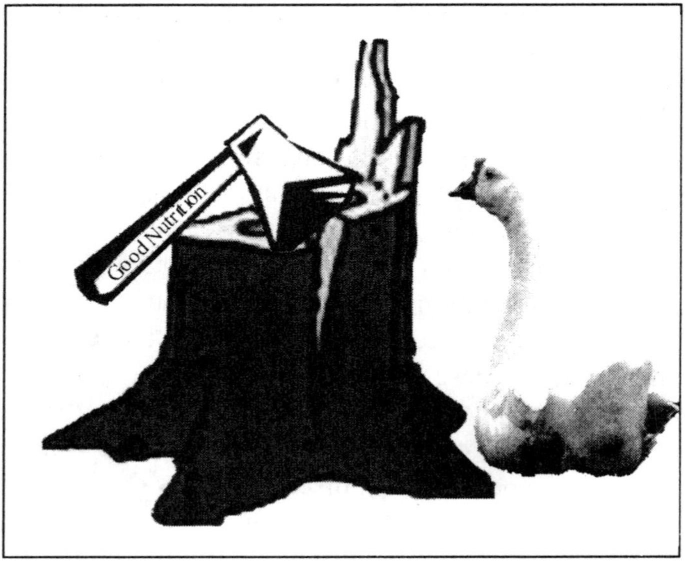

The evidence is quite clear, that with the billions of healthy domestic farm animals raised over the past half century, virtually free of most of these chronic diseases, good baseline nutrition has been preventive for the chronic diseases. Prior to their complete and balanced diets, many domestic animals experienced chronic diseases, and those lacking good nutrition today also frequently experience various non-infectious, chronic diseases. It is very rare among the animals to see calves with six legs, two tails or two heads. For a good review of the types of birth defects experienced before good nutritional practices were implemented, I recommend you review the book Nutrition and Physical Degeneration. (37)

The source/cause of the majority of non-infectious, chronic diseases, I propose, is due to malnutrition, affecting the body's ability to effectively build and maintain the connective tissues.

Chapter 6

Connective Tissue Disorder (CTD).

The cause alleged for most non-infectious, chronic diseases

It is undeniable that:

1. Connective tissues, collagen and elastin, provide the basic support structure for the body of humans and all other animals.
2. Collagen is to animals as cellulose is to plants, such as fruits, cereal grains and vegetables.
3. The Connective tissues represent twenty five percent (25%) of the protein found in the body.
4. The connective tissues consist primarily of the amino acids proline and lysine, but other amino acids are involved, such as glycine and a number of other chemicals that are necessary in the assimilation and repair of these tissues.
5. Proline is found in greater abundance in animal tissues, with beef and pork containing significantly more than is found in poultry meats like chicken and turkey.

The lack of the right chemicals in the diet to produce and/or maintain these tissues, gives rise to what I shall call "Connective Tissue Disorder,"

(CTD). I have not found this disorder listed in the medical journals, nor on the internet. However, I believe it is so pervasive in the human population that it is the most likely cause of up to seventy-five percent of the non-infectious, chronic diseases.

Consider the fact that connective tissues are found in every cell of the body. CTD is nothing more, or less, than deterioration of the connective tissues. The most probable cause for this deterioration is the lack of the amino acids and other chemicals in the diet that would allow the body to make the needed repairs as the tissue wears out. This is called malnutrition! It was once claimed that the body replaces itself about every seven years, provided that it has the appropriate nutrients to do so.

The specific location of the deterioration will vary over time, and can occur anywhere in the body. The deterioration will not occur instantly, but would be a slow process, possibly taking years, depending on the extent of malnutrition experienced. The location of the deterioration will determine the name of the resulting chronic disease. For instance, if the elastic covering on the outside of all arteries is deteriorating, this weakness in the artery will cause a bulge to form when it becomes weak enough and gives way under elevated blood pressure surges. This would be called an aneurysm. If the problem occurs in the elastic inner lining of the artery, a rough spot will form, called a lesion or plaque. Over time, this could cause blockage of the artery. The material actually doing the blocking could be any material normally transported throughout the body, within the circulatory system, such as white cells, red cells, platelets, fibrin, or cholesterol. The actual *cause* of the blockage would be none of these materials. So, if one is to prevent arterial blockages, it is essential to prevent the deterioration of the connective tissue lining the arteries.

This also applies to the elastic tissues in the wall of the stomach or other parts of the digestive tract, the lungs, the nerve insulators throughout the nervous system, the bones throughout the body and the connective tissues providing the cushion between all joints. And those are only <u>some</u> of the possibilities!

Such deterioration gives rise to chronic diseases, including various forms of cancer, arthritis, and the many neurological diseases that are becoming all too common. I estimate that no less than seventy-five percent (75%) of the non-infectious diseases are caused by CTD.

The major components of the body that concern me in this chapter, deal with the actual support structures that enable a person to stand, walk, perform work or exercise, and carry out the activities essential for normal movement and function.

The bones in the body provide the basic support for standing erect, moving about as we get up or sit down, driving a car or any other activities associated with normal body movement. Additionally, they protect the organs from physical harm caused by outside sources such as a fall or accident.

The muscles also play a role in their ability to do work. One must realize however, that each muscle fiber, each muscle bundle and each whole muscle contains a protective covering, giving strength and stability to each muscle fiber. This covering protects the muscles from rupture, provided that the integrity of the connective tissues is in tact. In some instances though, one may stretch or overload the muscle beyond the elastic limit and we say we have pulled a muscle or a tendon.

It has been alleged that statin medications used to lower cholesterol have impaired the maintenance or rebuilding of the connective tissues protecting the muscles. This causes the patient to lose the ability to stand or walk, because of the weakness in the muscles or the protective connective tissues.

Let me reemphasize that all structures within the body have a protective cover or internal support system consisting of connective tissues.

Much like the muscles, the cover provides elasticity and resistance to rupture. Red blood cells must be carried throughout the body without rupturing in order to deliver the oxygen and other nutrients essential to life. The lungs, stomach, and nervous system must all have the elasticity to expand and contract if we are to breathe normally, move the foods through the digestive system and eventually eliminate the waste products. The nervous system must have some elasticity to stretch rather than break as we move our bodies in work or exercise.

Connective tissues, collagen and elastin, are the materials most essential for ensuring sufficient elasticity to meet these needs. The basic structure of bones is collagen. The bones, as they develop are soft and pliable. As the matrix of collagen is formed, it is later hardened by the influx of calcium, phosphorus, magnesium and other chemicals. This provides the strength necessary for the bones to do their job.

There are several classes of collagen, depending upon the animal species. They are made of strings of amino acids that are twisted like a rope with two or three strands making each protein. There are two unique amino acids: proline and lysine that are subsequently converted to a less soluble form known as hydroxyproline and hydroxylysine. These amino acids, found in collagen proteins, are not found in any other proteins. The strands of collagen have a very high tensile strength. It is greater than steel! Other amino acid strands used to make other types of protein, are not as strong. Through cross linking and hydrogen bonding some types and sources of collagen are made stronger and more elastic.

Elastin, the protein found most often in the tendons of animals, is found throughout the body and is formed by compacting collagen fibers more densely and through additional cross linking of the fibers. The elastin becomes much stronger and less soluble than normal collagen. Neither collagen nor elastin is easily solubilized, nor do enzymes readily destroy the fibers.

Collagen is very unique in that it is only found in animal tissues. However, the quality and strength differs significantly between the various animal species. The larger the animal, the stronger the collagen and elastin must be, to support and protect the larger organs.

The skin of all animals is the largest organ in the body. A healthy animal will have skin that is pliable and elastic. The thickness will vary depending upon the protective role needed for any specific part of the body. The sole of the feet, the back, and the palms of one's hands are less elastic and tougher than say the abdominal area, the flank, or neck tissue where the skin is more pliable, more elastic and thinner. In addition to protecting the internal organs from outside forces, the skin serves to block bacteria and other harmful things from entering the body. It permits the elimination of fluids by perspiration which provides a cooling effect for the body.

The recommendations of the HOD make it quite apparent that they have little or no concern for the composition or function of the basic support structure of the body. They appear to care even less about the contributions to be made by the many different foods. The old saying "You can't make a silk purse from a sows ear" is still true. By the same token, you can't repair or replace the damaged or worn out connective tissues with the chemicals present in celery stalks or asparagus spears. These chemicals are to be found in animal source foods, such as beef and pork.

There is much that has been known about the human body for at least sixty years: This includes its chemical composition, how the various organs function, the chemicals that it manufactures, and the various sources of foods that can provide proper nourishment for the body to be complete and balanced (healthy).

If a complete and balanced diet is not fully achieved, one is almost assuredly going to experience one or more of the over one thousand non-infectious, chronic diseases known to man. In an unhealthy state (malnourished), one is also more susceptible to contracting one or more of the infectious diseases.

The elderly and the young are always cautioned to get their flu shot or other vaccinations because they are at higher risk. In other words, they are likely to be malnourished due to their dietary habits.

The medical uses of collagen:

Collagen is used to repair arterial systems that are bulging with aneurisms. This collagen is normally taken from a fraction of pig collagen. Of course, the cost is quite high by the time it's been processed and purified, and made into a patch or a stent, or used as an injection.

Collagen injections are used for cosmetic purposes, to reduce wrinkles. Unfortunately, the fix for cosmetic purposes is temporary, because it is eventually absorbed by the body.

I believe we would be better off consuming a higher level of good collagen in our diet, rather than buying it as medical devices. We cannot rely on fruits, vegetables or soy protein to supply these essential chemicals in adequate amounts for maintaining the connective tissues throughout the body.

Chapter 7

You Have a Right to Good Health

Why don't more people have it?

Essentially, good health is freedom from all diseases. This does not negate the need to see the health professional for the annual check-up. Most people are unaware of the joy of good health until they get sick. When they recover, they quickly forget how miserable it was to be sick. You are the one who cares the most about your health. After all, if you don't care, who will?

"Our bodies are apt to be our autobiographies." ~Frank Gillette Burgess

Many individuals abuse their bodies by choice, using alcohol, drugs, tobacco, foods in excess and lack of exercise. Knowingly, they do not consume a healthy diet, including a good multivitamin and mineral supplement. Unfortunately, most individuals that I have interviewed over the past five years do not have the slightest understanding of how to build and maintain good health.. Most people believe the food pyramids, food guidelines, and other recommendations from the HOD have to be true, but most of the time they lose because it isn't:

- I would estimate that more than eighty percent (80%) do not take a good supplement based upon the RDA's

- An equal or greater number fear eggs, beef, pork, butter, milk and other dairy products because of their belief that these foods will cause heart attacks, strokes, and plugged arteries due to fat and cholesterol.
- A large number, due to these fears, have become vegetarians, avoiding meat, milk, and eggs.
- In search of better health, a very large number have bought into the constant barrage of nutritional information and studies that are reported on the radio infomercials, in the news papers, and on television. Many of these reports are from the most prestigious universities, government laboratories, medical research foundations, and those who market a wide variety of supplements with little or no substance to support their claims.
- To be healthy, one must think well beyond foods and supplements. About twenty factors are reviewed in detail in Book II of this series that, if followed, will lead to a more perfect health.

- Taking control of your health is essential to achieving good health. and sustaining it for a lifetime.

I dare say that most people go to the doctor to get healthy. **What a mistake!** That is <u>not</u> the business of a physician. They are in the business of healing, not prevention, cure, or making a person healthy! If you have an accident or an infectious disease, they can diagnose the nature of the illness and provide medications, surgeries and/or care. They have done a good job of preventing and curing many of the infectious diseases.

However, preventing or curing chronic diseases is counter to their business needs. If patients did not have chronic diseases, they would lose about seventy-five percent (75%) of their business. Could this be the reason they treat the symptom, but not the cause? I have asked many physicians why they do not determine the nutritional status of their patients. Those who answer the question have told me that there is no money in nutrition! Indeed, I believe that a person can experience good health for about a dime a day for their nutritional supplements. (See Book II of this series).

The HOD provides all manner of pain medications but will seldom, if ever eliminate the cause, except by surgery. There is abundant evidence that many of these medications have very dangerous side effects that can damage one or more organs such as the kidney, or liver.

A good example of this is arthritis. They provide pain medications, steroid injections, and joint replacements; however, I have never seen any technical articles that suggest recommendation that would prevent the onset or cure of the disease. Nutrition is virtually never mentioned.

Most people fail to achieve and maintain good baseline nutrition because of the many erroneous recommendations by the HOD that has instilled fear of many good foods. Neither do they understand what vitamins and minerals they should include in their daily diets. Instead of taking a well balanced multivitamin and mineral supplement that adequately protects their health, people frequently choose to select two or three individual vitamins believing they have protected their health. If you want to ensure that your diet contains adequate trace minerals, don't rely on foods consumed to provide them.

Chapter 8

Hospital Practices and Policies

Why a hospital may be worse than the disease — the "Patient's Bill of Rights" is being destroyed.

I don't think anyone wants to go to the hospital, but there are times when it is the best thing that could happen. What you need to know is that with the changes in administrative policies and practices, the hospitals have caused the Patient's rights to be in real danger, and *caution is advised*!

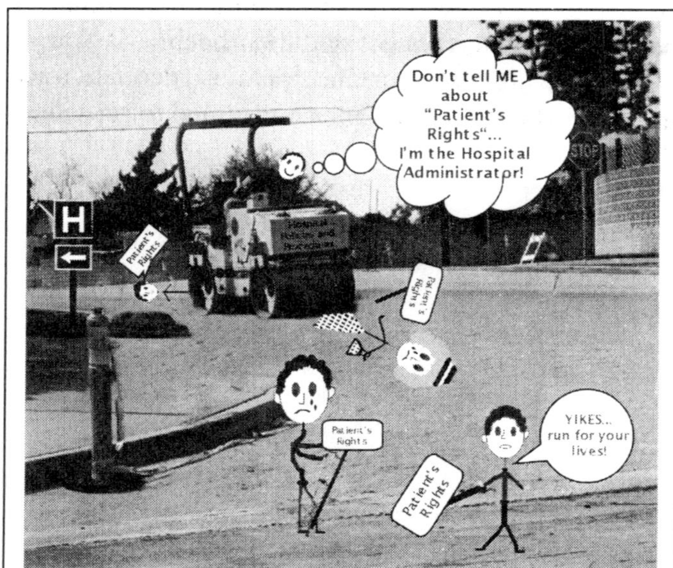

Practices that place the patient in harms way

Many of the incidents that I refer to here are reported in the news media. Some have been first hand incidents involving myself, friends and family members.

In order to help protect a loved one while in the hospital, our family decided the only way was to provide around the clock surveillance, to observe the patient's condition, and to help ensure the accuracy of medications being given. Why is this necessary? There are numerous factors entering into the equation, making the likelihood of mistakes certain without such surveillance.

One institution seeking physicians to work in their facilities has described what they expect from physicians, if they are to have a profitable and successful practice. They would expect the physician to maintain a client base of 2,000 patients with the addition of 30-45 new patients each month to make up for the loss of patients, due to death or relocation. With this patient load, mistakes will invariably happen.

- Add to that the occasional lack of competence of some practitioners
- Their hiring of staff (Nursing professionals) with minimal training
- Hiring staff, that is not fluent in the English language, giving rise to numerous mistakes
- In the medical care business, any mistake can be life threatening!
- Lowered standards of sanitation practices
- Lowered standards for safety practices
- Lowered standards for maintenance
- Lowered standards for quality assurance

The practices cited above have been causal in numerous deaths, increased pain, costs, and disabilities that could have been avoided.

It was reported recently, that a patient in an Anaheim hospital was accidentally given a transfusion of the wrong blood type, resulting in the patient's death.

In another recent situation, a patient in a North Orange County hospital was experiencing difficulty. The daughter, who was by her side attempted to call the nurse. Unable to get a response, one of the sanitation workers searched the floor of the hospital to find the floor nurse, but none were currently on the floor. She did locate a physician who immediately went to the room. While the physician was standing in the doorway, the patient died from chocking, as he tried to reach a nurse to help perform a "Code Blue." We have all heard of incidents where the wrong kidney was removed, or the wrong limb was cut off. This occurs all too often, and I believe these mistakes are due to the above mentioned practices.

I found some very disturbing information in my medical files during a recent stay in a hospital. While reviewing the admission summary, I observed that it was noted that I had a history of hypertension and hyperlipidemeia. The hypertension was accurate, but the hyperlipidemeia was without basis. The physician, when confronted on the matter, advised me that I had a long term problem with high cholesterol. At the time, my cholesterol was 134 mg and had never been over 174 mg to my knowledge. He was claiming that it had been over 200 mg. He said he would provide the source information for his diagnosis, but never did so. Why is this of importance? The statin drug he was prescribing for this non existent problem is known to have major adverse side effects. If I were applying for health insurance or life insurance, it would likely cost more or would not be available. If I were seeking a job, I might be denied because of his erroneous diagnosis.

In another situation, a patient who was in the hospital for a hip replacement was similarly misdiagnosed. According to their records she weighed 189 pounds. With a height of 5' 6 1/2in., she would have a body mass index of 30. The range for obesity is from 30-40 BMI. Morbid obesity is from 40-50. She was barely in the obese range at 30. The doctor constantly made references in her records that she was morbidly obese. For morbid obesity she would have had to weigh 252 – 300 pounds! Such a misdiagnosis could affect insurance cost, or employability. Why would he do this? This same patient, previous to entering the hospital, had been declared a non-diabetic. During her stay following surgery, she was routinely given IVs to prevent dehydration. The IV was a dextrose (sugar) solution. After each liter of solution, they tested her blood for sugar, only to find it elevated. This called for an insulin injection to lower the sugar in her blood. This cycle of dextrose followed by insulin was continued for several days. When I questioned this absurd practice, the RN checked with the doctor. It was changed to saline solution instead of dextrose. This significantly reduced the need for insulin; however, when she left the hospital she had been diagnosed as a diabetic. Three years later, she is required to take medication for type II diabetes and remains diabetic. There seem to be no logical reason for putting a patient through this, except to support the sale of dextrose and insulin. What would be best for the patient?

During a recent hospitalization, I had the misfortune of seeing what *greed* really looks like and it is ugly! In this particular incident, the patient had seen the orthopedic surgeon for about a year. She had exhausted all available pain medications, as they caused internal bleeding. The doctor suggested the next step would be cortisone injections in the hip to relieve pain. The first shot gave relief for a few months but the second lasted much less. At that time the doctor recommended hip replacement surgery, and the patient agreed. During the pre-operation appointment, the patient was adamant about her problems with pain medications, and reported that even a baby aspirin every other day had caused internal bleeding.

The patient was asked to participate in a new drug test with an experimental blood thinner. Realizing that physicians can make more money conducting experimental studies, the patient thought perhaps better service would be provided if she agreed to the test. She was assured that the doctor understood that she did not want to be given aspirin, and that the test drug would only be given if conditions warranted.

The patient entered the hospital, a large hospital in North Orange County, and the surgery went as expected with the patient being taken to her room at 11:00 AM. Other than nausea, the patient appeared to be doing well as of 9 PM.

At 8:00 AM the next day, upon returning to the hospital, the patient was receiving a transfusion which suggested internal bleeding was ongoing. The floor nurse was called, to learn what was going on. She checked the records which confirmed that the patient had received a 325 mg aspirin in the recovery room, which she informed me, was an oversight on the part of the surgeon, who always orders aspirin in recovery. This was in spite of the warning bracelet that showed the patient reacted to aspirin.

The surgeon was called and at 11:00 AM he arrived, and entered into a heated discussion with the RN, telling her to give aspirin as ordered, saying that many patients believe they are allergic to things when they aren't. She said that it was her patient too, and refused to give further aspirin. The doctor told me that he had only given her one aspirin, and left the scene!

The patient continued to deteriorate for several days, losing five pints of blood (only two were replaced), becoming immobile from the loss of blood which caused a major blood clot in the leg that subsequently broke away and entered the lungs. This was diagnosed as possible pneumonia, and went untreated for two days. They then advised the family for two days that the patient might not make it through the night.

Fortunately, a pulmonary specialist was brought onto the case and in less than five minutes he had diagnosed the problem as blood clots. One clot in the leg extended from the knee to the groin. He informed the patient that she had experienced a meteor shower of small clots to the lungs. He took over the case, and gradually dissolved the clots with appropriate medications, which took about six months. This was six months of fear, never knowing if another clot would break away causing death or permanent disability.

To my surprise upon reviewing the records, there was no longer evidence that aspirin had been given. However, the experimental blood thinner had been administered at 7:00 AM; twenty four hours post surgery as ordered by the surgeon.

A review of the Prescriptive Instructions by the manufacturer of the experimental blood thinner revealed the following:

1. The experimental medication was contra-indicated, which means that it should not be given to females over 65 years of age. (Patient was 69 years at the time)

2. The medication should not be given to patients with hypertension. (Patient was on medication for hypertension)

3. This medication should not be given to patients with a history of bleeding. (Patient had several years' history of bleeding when taking pain medications, a fact the doctor knew about)

These factors alone should have eliminated the patient from the study!

4. Medication should not be administered to patients with aspirin in their body. (At 11:00 AM the surgeon believed the patient had aspirin in her system, whether she did or not)

5. Medication *should not* be administered to a patient *who is actively bleeding*. (Medication was administered at 7:00 AM at which time *the patient was receiving a blood transfusion*)

What could the surgeon be thinking? Could it have been the financial motivation to receive the $1,500-$5,000 fee paid by the drug manufacturer for the patient being in the test program? Was the physician willing to risk this patient's life for this meager amount of money?

Hip replacement surgery is said to cost around $35,000 in the U.S. In this instance, the hospital charges were $133,000 for the 17 days, rather than the 4-5 days that had been projected by the surgeon. In my opinion, such practice should not be allowed anywhere in the world. Should you or a loved one be considering a surgical procedure; then please:

1) Think twice, and check the prescriptive instructions before agreeing to any experimental test program for the new drug.

2) I have been authorized to release a copy of the hospital records pertaining to the above case for those who may be selecting an orthopedic surgeon in North Orange County.

Policies that usurp the "Patient's Bill of Rights"

When mistakes are made in hospitals, there is little doubt that contributing to the mistakes, are the policies that have been implemented across the country in many hospitals. These policies restrict the patient's rights while providing a greater financial return to the hospitals and physicians.

- When entering the Emergency Room, the admitting physician virtually takes control of your life. He refers other physicians onto the case, solely at his discretion. It doesn't matter if you have insurance that permits you to choose your physician you are at the mercy of the admitting physician, a house physician. I believe a patient should have the right to choose a specialist. One that they have been paying for through their insurance, and not be forced to rely on a house physician, whose competence could not compare to that of a specialist! Yes, the hospital makes more money when they control the physician as a house physician, rather than one who is authorized to practice in the hospital, but is an independent physician.

  It is indeed difficult to obtain the services of one's Primary Care Physician, or other specialist, under these circumstances. There appears to be Policies, written and unwritten, that precludes your physician from entering the hospital, without their being referred by the admitting physician, who is very reluctant to make such referrals. These policies are destroying the careers of many good physicians by making it difficult for them to adequately serve their patients. Through these policies, they have an adverse effect on the physician's income as well, by way of their manipulations.

What can be done to change these practices and policies?

1. If there are laws that require proper training, experience, levels of sanitation, and all of the other problems that exist under current practices — they should be enforced.
2. The patient should be able, if they can pay for it, to have their physician of choice, provided that the physician is qualified to practice in the facility where the patient is located.
3. If there are no laws to prevent the violations of the patient's rights, then it is clearly time for new legislation.
4. The fourth, and most likely to be effective, would be a class action lawsuit to get their attention, hitting them in the pocket book where it hurts!

Chapter 9

Are You in Control of Your Health – or is the HOD?

Delegation to the HOD is not an option!

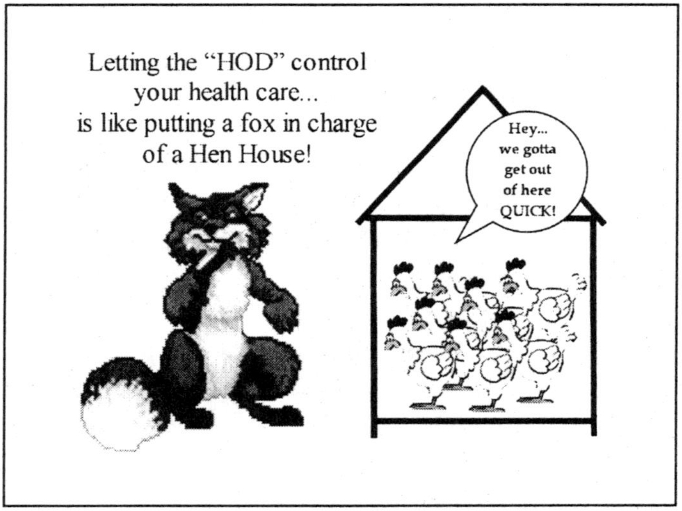
Letting the "HOD" control
your health care...
is like putting a fox in charge
of a Hen House!
Hey...
we gotta
get out
of here
QUICK!

If you are reading this book, you have already received the greatest gift you will ever receive in this life, and that is *the gift of life itself*. What you choose to do about protecting it is your decision. Protecting your life by protecting your health is, or should be, in your control.

As Yogi Berra, the famous baseball player once said:

"When you come to a fork in the road, take it".

This Series of books is being written so that you can make informed decisions when you choose that fork in the road. The information you will need to achieve a more perfect health is in Book II of this Series.

However, you need to know the degree to which some will go, in order to make a buck as well as try to control your health.. Bear in mind that I said, "to control your health" and not to make you healthy. There are many individuals who are more interested in your money than your good health, no matter what they say. What they say can sometimes be very convincing, and thus must be put to the test of common sense.

Control of your health is your responsibility! This requires <u>you</u> to make many decisions as you go through life.

- What foods to eat?
- When to eat?
- How much to eat?
- Should I take vitamin supplements, and which ones, how much, when?

"The patient should be made to understand that he or she must take charge of his own

life. Don't take your body to the doctor as if he were a repair shop". ~Quentin Regestein

There are literally hundreds of decisions to make. How well you answer these questions will dictate to a large extent, how healthy you will be.

Your physician or other health professional should **only** be there to advise or recommend what you could or should be doing. The decision and control should be in your hands. Whether or not you heed their advice in taking a particular medication or having a particular surgical procedure done is up to you. I have some very specific recommendations for you to consider when making your decisions in health matters:

- When a medication is recommended, take the time to consult the literature available from the manufacturer as well as other sources, to become fully knowledgeable of the various known side effects. In most instances a more legible and I believe complete disclosure, can be found on the manufacturer's web site or at sites such as drugs.com or Medline.com. I have found some instances where the pharmacy's or manufacturer's disclosures are less complete than one found on the suggested internet sites. The manufacturer's disclosure for medication for one patient interviewed was prescribed for hypertension, failed to declare that the medication could reduce sex drive but this side effect was disclosed on the internet site. Therefore, one cannot be too cautious when confirming potential side effects from various drugs — you can control this!

- Take the time to find out where the professional studied. Ask what subjects were actually in the areas of expertise they are advising you on. If they are advising you on diets, foods, or supplements, did they in fact study this area of science? A number of universities, such as UC Irvine do not teach a single course in nutrition, and others offer it as an elective, so they may have very limited knowledge concerning nutrition. I have a friend whose physician recommended supplements costing him $400 per month. There is much evidence that $3.50 per month will provide all the supplements you need and would likely be safer for you. *Your money, your decision!*

- *Professionals who speak with the "one voice" of the HOD — Telling you to* avoid animal fats, foods containing cholesterol, drink only low or no fat milk, eat no more than one egg per day, discourage an RDA type multi vitamin and mineral supplement, follow the food pyramid and the food guidelines, etc., *should be replaced with a competent, thinking professional, who is capable of searching for the truth and, hopefully, is more concerned about your health than his or her paycheck!*

You are the one who can control the condition of your health. It is your choice to eat certain foods, to take medications, and decide if you want to take a vitamin and mineral supplement. In other words, you have no one to blame but yourself! The HOD can recommend all manner of things, but you make the decisions. With this approach, you can never be their prey. One by one the people in this country can take charge of their health, and, I believe, avoid many of the non-infectious, chronic diseases. On an individual basis, I believe you can take control of your health and you can win your war against the HOD.

How will this benefit you?

- Reduce the visits to your doctor except for annual physicals or to get treatment for infectious diseases.
- Reduce the cost of medications related to chronic diseases
- Reduce the need for surgeries.
- Reduce the costs for hospital or other medical care
- In turn, this should reduce the financial burden on Medicare and/or insurance companies which over the long term, should result in lower insurance costs, and lower taxes.

- Better quality of life — the greatest benefit!

"He who enjoys good health is rich, though he knows it not." ~ Italian Proverb

The objective in taking charge of one's own health does not mean that you become your own physician and self medicate. You are the one that has the most to gain by being healthy, and indeed, your health service providers have the most to lose if you are healthy. With respect to the non-infectious, chronic diseases, you have the power and the ability to control the status of your health. No one is likely to care more about your good health than you. In my opinion, the HOD could not care less about your being healthy. Their concern appears to be with diagnostics, treatment and care. That leaves you with the responsibility for prevention and cure when it relates to the non-infectious, chronic diseases.

The HOD has virtually divorced itself from the field of nutrition. Many of the physicians with whom I have spoken have told me that they have no interest in nutrition simply because there is no money in it. Common sense will be your greatest weapon in this battle if you are to win and be healthy. Identifying and selecting qualified health. care professionals is one of your big challenges, whether it is your physician, surgeon, nurse, personal trainer, dietitian, nutritionist, or any other specialist.

The first priority is to confirm that the individual selected is technically qualified and competent in his or her chosen field of work. Second, the person should have unquestionable integrity.

Consider the selection of an auto mechanic to service your new $60,000 SUV. Most owners would not take it to a mechanic who could not support his or her claims of certified training to properly service your particular model of vehicle. That speaks to competence, but what about integrity?

I am reminded of an instance a few years ago when I took my car to the dealership to have the air conditioning system serviced. I was told that the compressor was out, and the cost to repair would be about $650. This appeared high, so I took the car to a non-dealer shop that had a good reputation for competence and ethics. The mechanic took one look and informed me that before he could diagnose any problem with the system, he would have to replace a bearing on the compressor that was frozen. Upon replacing the bearing at a cost of $25, the rest of the system worked fine. I asked how the dealer service personnel could have made their diagnosis, and he told me that they couldn't!

I feel certain that most people have had similar experiences. These incidents, when they happen, do not usually represent a life and death situation — just a loss of money.

Let's say that instead of an SUV, you have a private Jet. Would your selection of a mechanic be a little more stringent than for your SUV? Preventive maintenance should certainly have a very high priority. Fixing the problem, or cure, is exceedingly important as well, lest you fall from the sky and die from the crash.

So, what does all this have to do with health anyway? The new SUVs have been built with computers, numerous safety devices, hi-tech engines, transmissions and stabilizer systems. Such a sophisticated vehicle cannot compare with the complexities to be found in a personal jet aircraft. Even more important is the fact that the complex jet would be like a cheap toy when compared with the human body.

Animals, including humans, are essentially complete factories which can, when provided with the proper raw materials, produce the hormones, antibodies, enzymes, proteins, amino acids, red and white blood cells, muscle, bone, the nervous system, as well as every cell in the body. It can repair itself by removing the worn out cells and replacing them with new cells and can destroy many of the invading bacteria, viruses, and other micro organisms that cause diseases. Compared to an expensive SUV or Jet Plane, the human body is a ***priceless*** machine, and certainly deserves a professional who has more concern than appears to be had by most individuals in today's world of medicine.

Learn the truth about health and nutrition

A critical review of the recommended references listed in the back of this book can provide a more balanced perspective on what constitutes the truth regarding the controversial subject of animal fats and cholesterol (See Appendix A). I find these references to be quite accurate.

My primary opposition is related to *the "one voice" position* of those in the HOD. It reflects a lack of open mindedness, and a gross lack of scientific curiosity on the part of many in the HOD. They seem to accept the contrived myths as though they represent the absolute truth. This reflects a herd mentality.

When reviewing news articles on health, <u>regardless of their source</u>, I consider first what their agenda might be. Are they selling a product or service or is it reflective of an unbiased research. study? Has the work been duplicated by other researchers in the field studied? All too often the agenda is to sell products and/or services. The unwitting individuals, who never question it, are easily caught in their snare.

Serious questions should be asked when considering any recommendation from those in the HOD. The first question that I would ask you is: *Has your health care professional taken the necessary action to ensure that you are free from nutritional deficiencies?* In my opinion this should be the first step in achieving "a more perfect health". If your health professional is concerned with, and promoting, the concepts put forth by the HOD then I recommend you find a professional with an open mind, and the curiosity to learn the truth with respect to nutrition. This is especially true for those who learned their skills subsequent to 1965. By then, the books had already been changed to include the fat and cholesterol myths, as well as the various other recommendations designed to cause people to have a higher incidence of chronic diseases.

Good baseline nutrition ensures that all known vitamins, minerals, essential fatty acids, essential amino acids and other nutrients are being met by your dietary program. This will:

- Make it possible for you to avoid many if not all of the chronic diseases.
- Make it possible for your health care professional to more accurately diagnose and treat your problem(s) successfully.

It has been my experience that the individual who sustains good baseline nutrition will have far fewer needs to see the health care professional for diagnosis and/or treatment of the chronic diseases.

Supplements that I think one should take

We should all be taking a supplement that includes approximately thirty chemicals. There are a few products on the market that **try** to meet that. They get a little side-tracked at times trying to hype the product and sales, therefore, profits, at the expense of the truth. Even the best of them are subject to those pressures.

I believe though, that you need to have such a supplement with your biggest meal of the day, if you take one a day, and that **is** my recommendation. If you are under serious stress or have been mal-nourished for some period of time, two or even three tablets a day, for brief periods would provide very low risk. It is really more an insurance policy than anything else, if you're getting a good diet. Otherwise, it's not something that would hurt you. It's not something that costs a lot of money, but it sure is effective, if your diet does not include all of the trace minerals and vitamins known to be essential for complete and balanced nutrition.

This has been proven for twenty-five to fifty years with domestic pets and farm animals. I believe that humans have similar genetic makeup, including good genes, and they can be as healthy as the other animals.

The philosophy that I follow, and recommend, has been responsible for billions of healthy animals. How about your philosophy?

You'll note that throughout this book, there are some areas relating to health and nutrition that I haven't mentioned. And the reason that I haven't, is that I'm not recommending any of those products. I have absolutely no faith in them. I'm talking about natural, organic, herbal, and similar concepts. You see, it's very simple. I know that there have been billions and billions of animals that were **very, very** healthy, free of chronic diseases, living healthy lives through **all** stages, by having diets formulated to the RDA.

I know a lot of people have been eating "organic" and "natural" and vegetarian — and it hasn't worked. Nor have the recommendations of the HOD worked.

You do not need "organically grown", "range" eggs, "free range" eggs or brown eggs over white eggs The people who are selling you those products would like you to believe that this is the panacea for all illnesses. If it were that good to have such products, the farmers would be feeding it to their animals — they don't, it is not cost effective.

I believe that though some of these diet programs work, the only measure of their success, is that they empty your pocket while filling theirs. Most of those selling vitamin-mineral supplements, at outrageous prices, are selling you much higher dosages than you would get from a good RDA type supplement. But the "mega-doses" will serve more to throw an imbalance in your diet, than to effect any improvement in your health.

So, stay away from them. They're over priced, they're multi-level marketed, or sold by way of infomercials. In my opinion, their formulas have generally been developed by way of focus group marketing techniques, or formulated based upon polling data. That's not the way to solve ones health problems. Stick with the tried and the proven, and like I say, billions and billions of animals have proven for many years, a half a century, that RDA supplements with good foods is all one needs. No one has ever bothered to tell you how simple it can be to be healthy.

The individuals who fail to sustain good baseline nutrition can expect to endure:

- More frequent office visits to health care professionals due to chronic diseases
- Poor quality of life
- Mobility restricted or lost
- Increased surgeries

- Increased costs for medical services of all kinds
- Shorter life span

"Our body is a machine for living. It is organized for that, it is its nature. Let life go on in it unhindered and let it defend itself, it will do more than if you paralyze it by encumbering it with remedies". ~
Leo Tolstoy

Chapter 10

Recommended Research Programs

When I look back on the past half century, it is difficult to be proud of being in the sciences. The corruption that has entered in has stripped many scientists of their desire for finding the truth.

It has become clear to me that through manipulation and deception, the HOD has gradually been ***taking the gold out of the golden years*** for millions of people.

This they have done by causing more people to have chronic diseases with erroneous recommendations, backed up by fear tactics. They have totally misguided us on good foods, and the need for using vitamin and mineral supplements to help ensure our good health..

The objective of the research recommendations presented in this chapter is to make it possible for you to ***put the gold back into your Golden Years!*** These recommendations deal with chronic diseases, or what I consider the "manmade diseases", caused by poor health choices, or flawed recommendations from the HOD.

"In order to change we must be sick and tired of being sick and tired".

~Author Unknown

The nature and type of research projects considered here could contribute great benefits for humanity. None of these research projects offers big financial incentives, and thus will never be carried out with our present system for selection.

Essentially all of the state universities, numerous government institutions and tax exempt organizations, (though publicly funded) enter into joint ventures with food companies, pharmaceutical companies and others in order to share in the financial benefits resulting from patents. This approach places major constraints on the nature of research projects that will get funding. Basically, projects that would offer the potential for improving the health of individuals, effectively and economically, are not of any importance unless they also offer financial opportunities for those institutions or researchers.

It will be much easier to prevent the chronic diseases, if we first identify the cause. With some luck, the knowledge to prevent the diseases may let us cure them as well.

Major areas of needed research include:

Connective Tissue Disorder (CTD).

A better understanding of the manner in which the body assimilates, maintains, and repairs the connective tissues relates to almost all of the non-infectious, chronic diseases. The relationship of the nutritional needs to ensure proper function for these tissues represents the greatest research opportunity — and the least financially rewarding for the HOD. The potential rewards for the U.S. population is beyond calculation in terms of pain, suffering or financial considerations.

This complex chemistry has, in very recent years, been studied primarily for the medical benefits gained from use in the cosmetic field. It is injected to reduce wrinkles or reconfigure facial features. This initial application was followed by using a class of collagen from pigs to provide stents or patches used for repair of arterial damage caused by blocked arteries or weakened arteries that result in aneurisms. The use of collagen has been extensively used with great success in the treatment of burn victims.

The benefits to be gained from a better understanding of the connective tissues, so that proper assimilation, maintenance, and repair can be achieved through better nutrition, would prevent many of the chronic diseases. I estimate that no less than seventy-five percent of chronic diseases are the result of CTD.

This type of research should prove beyond the shadow of a doubt, the absolute relationship of nutritional deficiencies, and the cause of these diseases. The non-infectious, chronic diseases are associated with all cells of the body including the many organs. The more common diseases in this category include:

1. arthritis
2. cancer
3. bone diseases
4. arterial diseases
5. neurological diseases
6. pulmonary diseases
7. skin diseases

8. digestive system diseases
9. blood diseases
10. muscle diseases

There are other syndromes and disorders that should be researched to gain a better understanding of how to prevent or possibly cure them. They include:

- **Obesity**

People are quick to blame genetics for this problem, and everyone searches for that silver bullet to make obesity go away. I have found no bullets, but I think something much better. No one factor will allow a person to sustain their desired weight.

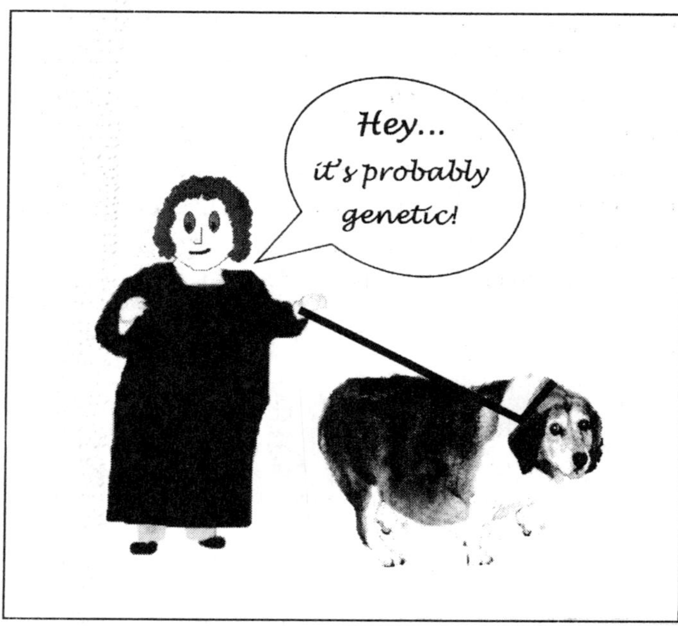

The relationship between complete and balanced diets, supported with multi vitamin and mineral supplements, while eating good foods and exercising in moderation seems a safer and less expensive approach than gastric by-pass surgery. Would it not be great if this hypothesis were confirmed? I know of individuals who have lost 175 pounds following similar practices.

- **Fluid retention and electrolyte balance**

I have observed many individuals with swollen arms and legs that truly reflect excess fluid retention. Though under the care of medical professionals for years, there seems to be nothing that rids them of this problem. I am advised that they are being *treated,* but not cured! Why? In this Twenty-first century do we not yet understand something so basic? The medical advertisements on TV will talk about various diseases, syndromes, or disorders, only to remind the viewer that there are treatments for this or that problem. They never talk about prevention or cure. I believe patients deserve more than just treatments. Further research could possibly rid patients of these problems. If the prevention or cure could be done through nutrition, it would not offer great financial rewards for the researchers, but would certainly save a lot of pain, and misery. It would also save money spent for treatments which appear to accomplish nothing, except to prolong the misery.

- **Comprehensive review of the RDA's**

We know very little of the nutritional benefits of the numerous chemicals in foods. A very comprehensive research program designed to find the truth, rather than to meet the agenda of a particular food company or class of foods, could lead to improved health for all individuals.

- **Bone deposition and depletion.**

Based upon the condition of the population in this country, there is clear evidence that we need to know a lot more of the basic metabolism of bone synthesis and what leads to loss of bone density. Many of the arthritic conditions are related to deterioration of cartilage between the bones. This could benefit from research. as well. It is commonly reported that 75 million individuals suffer from the various forms of arthritis.

- **Causes of Type II Diabetes**

If ever there was a man made disease, it has to be Type II diabetes. My belief is that the HOD recommendations, along with disregard for health. by individuals, gives rise to the growing number of individuals diagnosed as diabetic. A good research program to learn the basic truths as to the causes and the influence of complete and balanced nutrition on this disease will provide the answers as to how it can be prevented or cured.

▪ Causes of cancer related to nutrition

I believe there's a necessity for research. into the various *causes* of cancer. Only with such research are we likely to find avenues into prevention or cures. The CDC reported one of the cancers was thought to be due to the absence of an enzyme that contained pyridoxine. This clearly implicates nutritional deficiencies. Even if the new stem cell research were effective in doing repairs, it wouldn't be a long term benefit until you have ensured the base line nutrition of the individual.

▪ Blood Pressure. — Optimal Control

Blood pressure justifies a substantial study. This should be directed toward finding the optimal blood pressure, and the minimum that would always ensure that enough oxygen is being directed to the most distal parts, including the brain. Recent changes in the recommendations for blood pressure, lowering from 170/90 to 120/60 comes under question. Is this like the lowering of other standards — to create more patients?

There is a great opportunity for finding many of the answers regarding the cause of the non-infectious, chronic diseases. This, I believe, could be achieved with fairly simple, inexpensive research, compared to what's being done now. We simply need to look at the benefits to be derived from complete and balanced nutrition! What has been happening is that nutritional contributions to good health are being ignored, in order to find and exploit the benefits of medications and surgeries offering greater financial opportunities.

A program of research for each of the major systems in the body would be totally in order. The biggest project should be tied to the connective tissues. It could relate to multiple sclerosis, muscular dystrophy, aneurysms, blocked arteries, neurological diseases, irritable bowel syndrome, and the various forms of arthritis. Nearly every facet of the body is affected by the quality and condition of the connective tissue that supports each and every structure. It must be properly nourished and repaired on an ongoing basis to insure that the organs are protected, and that the tissues are properly supporting all of the organs, keeping the skin intact, keeping the arteries, veins, nerves, bronchial tubes, lungs and the brain all in fit condition, so that they are functioning in a healthy manner.

Chapter 11

Recommended Sources of Funding

With the billions spent each year on medical research. that is funded from donations, tax monies., and numerous companies, I believe the tax monies and donations should be redirected to those research areas which seek to identify the *cause* of chronic diseases, rather than new treatments via medications and surgeries.. The benefit is likely to be new found disease prevention saving countless dollars with the individuals incurring less pain and suffering.

To those philanthropic individuals who have been supporting the search for a *cure* for the non-infectious, chronic diseases over the past fifty years, I suggest you pay closer attention as to the type of research projects being funded from your contributions. If you stipulate the monies be invested in search of the *cause* of a disease, we are much more likely to be able to *prevent* the disease in the first place, and possibly provide the cure as well.

At this time, the total effort is being directed at finding a *cure* which is like finding the needle in a haystack. Such results have provided nothing more than new surgical techniques or dangerous medications for treatment of the symptoms. I believe it is inherently wrong to use taxpayer monies to identify new surgical techniques or medications. Leave this research to those who are profiting from these efforts. Let us find new ways to make the country healthier.

My real concern is that we have numerous tax exempt foundations for virtually any chronic disease that you could name. They are funding research. projects that are limited to a search for *cures*. They never give consideration to the possibility that the *cause* of a disease could be a more fertile field to search. Nor do they acknowledge any relationship to the nutritional status of the person with the disease, and possibly preventing or even curing the disease by providing complete and balanced nutrition. In all of the various organizations, tax exempt foundations, government organizations, private or public medical institutions, or any one else, I have not found any research that gives nutrition any possibility for holding the answers to the *cause* of non-infectious, chronic diseases.

We need research that results in improving the health. of people; this, in spite of the fact that it may not provide financial incentives sufficient to motivate manufacturers. The government spends taxpayer money in support of research. I believe these tax monies would be better directed at improving the health of the population. This could be accomplished by looking for the truth regarding the cause of diseases, especially where there is no financial incentive for research facilities to conduct such studies. Why should the taxpayers support the joint ventures of the universities with the pharmaceutical houses? Their interest is in the development of new medications that will generate tremendous profits. The taxpayer supported institutions should pursue the very important, but not necessarily financially rewarding research. We then would have the opportunity to find the cause or prevention of the chronic diseases — perhaps the cure!

Let us use taxpayer money to gain a better understanding of health issues, regardless of whether or not it makes money for the schools. This would reduce the potential for corruption of the researchers, and lessen the amount of "Junk Science". Prior to 1960 joint ventures were considered unethical. Companies could support university research at that time, but the researchers were allowed to publish their research, uncensored. Patents issued to government laboratories or universities were considered public property since the facilities were supported by taxpayer monies.

The pharmaceutical houses and food companies are businesses and have every right to make a profit from their investments in research.. However, they do not have the right to have the taxpayers fund their projects.

Chapter 12

Summary

The major points presented in this book were to inform you of the misconceptions that abound, with respect to the concepts for achieving good health. Non-infectious, chronic diseases have impacted the lives of almost every individual living in this country. The cost in terms of pain, suffering, loss of a quality life, loss of mobility, early death and the loss of loved ones, exceeds by far the financial losses that are associated with these diseases.

Chronic diseases are at their highest level in history, and more people are being afflicted with these diseases each and every day. The cost of medical care in the U.S., as reported recently in the Reader's Digest, are rising at twenty-five to thirty-two percent per year. In the year 2000, the CDC reported the total cost of medical services had exceeded one trillion dollars. In the Reader's Digest report, in April, 2006, the cost had reached two trillion dollars. (26) The CDC reported the cost for <u>infectious diseases</u>, and all types of accidents, the various forms of abuse associated with murders, robberies, domestic violence or other crimes, represented <u>twenty-five percent</u> of the total cost for medical care. That leaves <u>seventy-five percent due to chronic diseases</u>.

Six years later, in 2006, the costs of chronic diseases having doubled, are more like one and one-half trillion dollars!
Based upon the recent decisions to include obesity as a medical condition, thus qualifying gastric by-pass surgery for coverage by Medicare and the insurance companies means the total could continue it's inflationary pace. At a cost of twenty thousand dollars per surgery, and some physicians claiming to have performed one hundred thousand such surgeries, it becomes very costly. Unfortunately, it has been reported that around five percent (5%) of those having the surgery die within one year! Of those interviewed who had this surgery, two informed me they continued to have eating disorders even though each of them had six subsequent surgeries to fix the blockages caused by the failed surgery. Of the others interviewed who had the surgery, most complained of eating disorders of various types but had not elected for more surgeries to correct the problems. *The only thing they have proven with such surgeries is that the patients do lose weight!* Not all keep the weight off for a long time due to the ability of the stomach to expand over time, and many seem to regain their weight. There is a safer and better way to solve the problem of obesity, and that is with achieving, and maintaining, good baseline nutrition.

The Savings Account

Achieving good health is like setting up a savings account. The earlier you start it, the better the account will perform. The consistency of saving will ensure better performance as well.

So it is with your health account. You can start the account at any time, and it is never too late to start. The important thing is to get started and be consistent with your continual investment in the plan, in order to derive the greatest benefit, which is freedom from chronic diseases.

We must ask, what has gone wrong with the health. of humans? What appears to have gone wrong is that in the late 1950s to early 1960s that group, which I refer to as the HOD, did an about face regarding human nutrition!

The "one voice" recommendations from the HOD for humans since the late 1950s have been:

- Eat to the food pyramid
- Follow the food guidelines
- Avoid animal fats
- Avoid foods containing cholesterol
- You do not need multi vitamin or multi mineral supplements
- Eat lots of fruits and vegetables

This appears to be the cause for many of the chronic diseases found in humans. *Domesticated animals are not fed according to these recommendations and do not have the chronic diseases, except in rare instances if they become malnourished!* One can, on occasion, find other species of animals having the same chronic diseases observed in humans. This usually is found with domestic pets that have an imbalance in their diets due to too many table scraps or the feeding of non-balanced pet foods.

With the farmers, there is a financial incentive to have only healthy animals. This is achieved by providing complete and balanced nutrition using RDA type feed formulations. I have yet to talk with a farmer who feeds mega-dose vitamin supplements, exotic herbal chemicals with all of their nutritional claims, or any of the other supplements found in the ocean, the Black Forest, or distant Tibet.

Humans have a desire to be healthy; however, *there is no financial incentive for the medical professionals to have healthy patients.* **It is not good for business!** Their income is generated through diagnosing illness, treating the illness with medications or by surgeries, and providing the hospitalization or other forms of care. *Thus there is no interest in nutrition because there is no money in it.*

This position is clearly reflected in the breadth and depth of the research funded by the HOD. It is rare indeed for any of their research projects to consider even the possibility that nutritional deficiencies could play any part in causing the disease under study. Their programs refer to prevention concerns, but their actions deny any preventive research.

The majority of chronic diseases have been declared to have:

- No known cause
- No cure
- Require lifetime medications
- Require surgeries.

- Frequently require long term care

Who's the smartest of them all?

Each and every animal is indeed the most complex bag of chemicals ever known to man. It represents a complete factory that, when properly nourished, is programmed by way of the DNA to manufacture most of the chemicals needed to sustain your good health..

There are a few amino acids, (7 or 8) depending upon the species, and a couple of fatty acids that the body cannot produce, that are called essential. Of course, the body cannot produce the minerals or trace minerals that are so important in many of the billion or so chemical reactions that are reported to occur every day, so this is why I recommend the RDA type multi vitamin/mineral supplement to be taken daily with your main meal. The rest of all the chemicals can be manufactured from the foods consumed, provided there is proper nourishment going into the body via foods and supplements to ensure completeness and balance are provided.

It comes down to being smart, and there are an awful lot of physicians, scientists, nutritionists, dieticians and others, who apparently think they're quite smart, because they try to fine tune a system that they couldn't possibly begin to understand. There is no question in my mind, but that your body is far smarter, in knowing how to run the system, than any scientist or physician or nutritionist that you will ever meet.

You have to give it the opportunity to perform its functions and its jobs of converting the raw

materials that you feed it, into the chemicals that are essential to sustaining good health.

Will this really work for those who have experienced long term deficiencies? The best examples that come to mind were the POW's from WWII or Vietnam who were so emaciated when they were liberated or returned home. It took a while, but in time all the cases that I know of, appeared to make substantial recoveries from their malnourished state of health..

In painting a picture of health, one is better off to start with a big canvas and lay in the outline of the picture that you want to paint, and then gradually fill in more and more detail as you proceed. My philosophy is that we need to take a look at the big picture, look at the main support structures of the body and the main organs. To fully understand them before we get to the fine points of the finishing touches is the key to success.

The human body, or rather, the animal bodies in the animal kingdom, share the need for most of the same chemicals; the organs such as the liver, spleen, heart, pulmonary system, circulatory system, neurological system, bone structure, and the digestive system share comparable functions, and for the most part, the same metabolic processes, with similar enzymes, hormones, vitamins, minerals, physiological chemistry, and other chemical entities. It is the chemicals and functions that are very similar in spite of some physical differences between the species. The whole picture is exceedingly complex, with many interactions. Things are co-dependent, inter-dependent, whatever terms you want to use — it is complex and you can take any one little part out of context, so to speak, look at it under a microscope, and draw a totally erroneous conclusion, if that's all your study is based upon.

There are those who would like you to believe that achieving a healthy style of living, diet and nutrition are so complex, that no one could ever understand it. However, it is really quite simple, and I think the early scientists did a beautiful job, considering their tools available at that time in identifying the factors essential to good health..

I think this has been pretty well proven and is supported by the fact that upwards of at least 90% of the farm animals and 90% of the domestic pets are generally free of chronic disease; whereas, the human population is the reverse of that, with about 90% of them having one or more chronic diseases to deal with.

There are five areas where standards are being adjusted to increase the number of high risk patients. These standards are being adjusted by those individuals who are attempting to market medications, and/or surgeries. that would "control" the factors associated with:

- Hypertension (blood pressure standards)
- Type II diabetes (blood sugar standards)
- Obesity (standards for over weight, obese, and morbidly obesity)
- Coronary heart disease.
- Bone health. (calcium to phosphorous ratio)

Though my search of the literature has been exhausting, it has not been exhaustive. There are numerous areas where standards may have been artificially changed to create more patients that I am not aware of.

What concerns me about our future medical costs is the fairly new approach to nutrition within the HOD. That is, their reported desire to resolve nutritional problems by way of genetic manipulation. Common sense tells me — they don't have to do this with the farm animals, so why with humans? Unless good baseline nutrition is achieved and maintained, the gene repair would only be a stop-gap measure. Without good nutrition, the gene would be out of action in a short period of time. This type of treatment is not going to be cheap! Why do you think they choose this approach rather than recommending complete and balanced nutrition? (As with beef, pork, milk and eggs, along with a good RDA type supplement and a few fruits and vegetables.)

At this rate of increase in medical costs, there is little room for doubt that it will double again by the year 2010! *The following suggested course of action would reverse this trend limiting further increases. If only two-thirds of the population were to take charge of their health. through good nutrition, the total costs for medical services would be reduced by fifty percent (50%). The result would be a better quality of life with the money to enjoy it!*

It would be a bitter pill to take for those in the HOD, (No pun intended). If we don't do something, the financial burden will break the country. We must rid ourselves of these chronic diseases — and we must do it now!

The entire three hundred million people in the U.S. could collectively try to overcome this demonic presence in our society, and I predict they would lose! If we approach this on an individual basis, I predict that each and every one would win their war, simply by taking control of their health.

Your right to good health and freedom from manmade, chronic diseases is yours to claim! The manner in which this can be accomplished is beyond the scope of this book, but will be clearly presented in Book II which tells how you can achieve a more perfect health.

The main thing that sets humans apart from the rest of the animal species is choice! Now — the choice is yours! So…

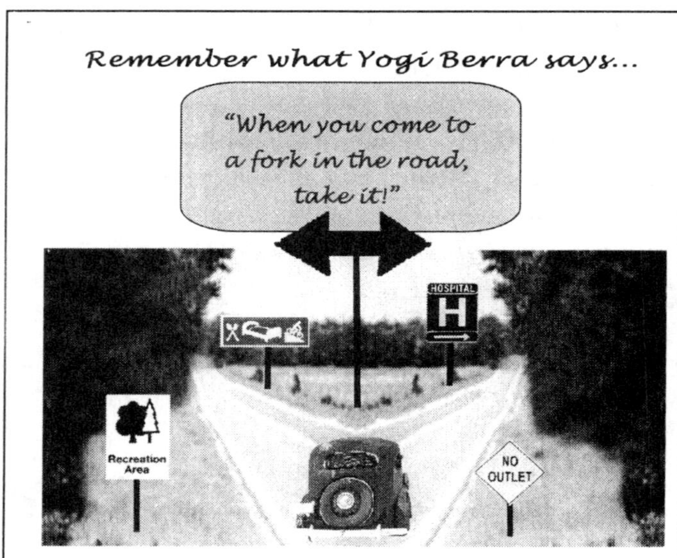
Remember what Yogi Berra says...
"When you come to a fork in the road, take it!"
HOSPITAL
H
Recreation Area
NO OUTLET

Biography

Background

I was born in 1931 at Doniphan, Missouri and grew up in the small farming community in the 1930's and 1940's. The town of Doniphan had 1600 inhabitants. I spent most of my after school hours working in the grocery store my father managed, learning about groceries, meats, and fresh produce.

I had a keen interest in the people of the community and their state of health.. At that time, most of the diseases were caused by bacteria such as diphtheria, polio, measles, mumps, malaria, rabbit fever, etc. The health of pets and farm animals caught my interest as well. It was exciting for me to see the changes in the health of humans and other animals as the nutritional developments of the 1940s were being implemented. The eggs no longer had soft shells; birth defects were less frequent among humans and the other animals. There were so few chronic diseases among the people, I considered them rare!

After graduating high school, I chose to attend college. This required about five and a half years for me to obtain the BS and MS degrees in the Food Science Department, at the University of Missouri. From there, I attended Michigan State University, earning a Ph.D. in Food Science & Nutrition in 1961.

My working career included three major food companies, where I conducted or directed others in, research. Early in my career, projects included product development, protein research, and other areas of applied research in food science and nutrition. Later, it included eight years of applied nutritional studies with domestic pets (dogs, cats, birds, and fish). The primary purpose of our research was to confirm through multi-generational studies that all products being marketed provided complete and balanced nutrition for all life cycles. This involved many breeds and weight ranges.

Five years ago, after several years of retirement, I became interested in obesity and the problems causing it. As I researched this problem, I came to believe that I knew the major cause, not only for obesity, but for the chronic diseases too. I arrived at my conclusions by pulling together information gleaned over the years relating to the animal kingdom, and the nutritional needs of the various species.

My goal in writing this series of books is to provide the opportunity for those interested, to make them selves more healthy through better understanding of the role that nutrition plays in their health.

Book I is directed at disclosing why so many people have chronic diseases and how to avoid them.

Philosophical Views on Health, Nutrition, and Chronic Diseases

The ever increasing incidence of chronic diseases among humans is alarming. when considering the fact that other animals have not experienced these same increases. What could be the cause for these differences? Other species of animals have, on occasion, incurred some of these diseases which are caused by malnutrition. The literature provides evidence of major changes that occurred in the late 1950s. These changes affected the manner in which nutritional research. was conducted. This resulted in a much different way of looking at nutrition and its effect on human health:

- Human nutrition was distanced from animal nutrition, although animal studies had earlier provided the foundation for human nutrition.
- The food pyramid.was developed and recommended increasing the consumption of fruits, vegetables, poultry meats, and soy protein. They eliminated beef and pork for thirty years, and severely limited milk and egg consumption.
- New recommendations discouraged the use of vitamin and mineral supplements.
- Animal fat was no longer to be consumed, but replaced with vegetable oils.
- Cholesterol was to be limited in the diet by avoiding beef, pork, milk, and eggs or other animal source foods.

- The scientific method for testing hypotheses was replaced with the double blind test using placebos.

These factors were designed to cause humans to experience chronic diseases due to malnutrition.

"The deviation of man from the state in which he was originally placed by nature seems to have proved to him a prolific source of disease." ~Edward Jenner

References

1. Alberts, Bray, Johnson, Lewis, Raff, Roberts, Walter, Collagen and Elastin, 1998 as cited in: www.garlandscience.com/ECB/about.html
2. Alzheimer's Foundation www.alz.org
3. Arthritis Foundation. www.arithritis.org
4. American Association for Cancer Research. (AACR) www.aacr.org
5. American Association of Hip and Knee Surgeons (AAHKS) www.mydna.com
6. American Cancer Society. www.cancer.org
7. American Dairy Science Association. www.adsa.org
8. American Diabetes Association. www.diabetes.org
9. American Dietetic Association. (ADA) www.eatright.org
10. American Egg Board. www.aeb.org
11. American Heart Association. www.americanheart.org
12. American Hospital Association. (AHA) www.aha.org
13. American Lung Association. www.lungusa.org
14. American Meat Institute. www.meatami.com
15. American Medical Association. www.ama-asn.org ,
16. American Medical Association, "United we triumph, divided we fail" 2003. www.ama-assn.org/ama/pub/article/1752-8219.html

17. American Osteopathic Association. www.osteopathic.org
18. American Poultry Association. www.amplyta.com
19. American Soybean Association. www.soygrowers.com , www.asasoya.org
20. American Stroke Association. www.strokeassociation.org
21. Centers for Disease Control and Prevention, (CDC). www.cdc.gov
22. Enig, Mary, Ph.D., and Sally Fallon, The Oiling of America, www.westonprice.org
23. Food and Drug Administration. www.fda.gov
24. Hawk, Philip B., Ph.D., Bernard L. Oser, Ph.D. and William H. Summerson, Ph.D., Practical Physiological Chemistry, 13th Ed., The Blakiston Company, N.Y., N.Y. 1954
25. Health Media of America and Somer, Elizabeth, M.A., R.D., The Essential Guide to Vitamins and Minerals, Harper Collins Publishers. 1992
26. Howley, Kerry I Can't Afford to Get Sick, Reader's Digest 91-99 April 2006
27. Johns Hopkins Family Health Book by The Johns Hopkins University Harper. Collins Publishers, Inc., New York, N.Y. 1999.
28. Mayo Clinic www.MayoClinic.com
29. Muscular Dystrophy Association. (MDA) www.mdausa.org
30. My Pyramid, www.usda.gov
31. National Academy of Sciences. www.nas.edu

32. National Dairy Council. www.nationaldairycouncil.org
33. National Heart, Lung, and Blood Institute. (NHLBI) www.nhlbi.nih.gov
34. National Institutes of Health. www.nih.gov, www.health.nih.gov www.grants.nih.gov/grants
35. National Multiple Sclerosis Society, www.nmss.org
36. National Research Council, Nutrient Requirements of Humans, 9th Ed. 1980
37. Price, Westin A., D.D.S., Nutrition and Physical Degeneration, 6th Ed., The Price-Pottenger Foundation, Inc., La Mesa, CA, 2004. www.ppnf.org
38. Ravnskov, Uffe, M.D., Ph.D., The Cholesterol Myths: Exposing the Fallacy That Cholesterol and Saturated Fat Cause Heart Disease. New Trends Publishing, Inc., Washington, D.C. 2000
39. Ravnskov, Uffe, M.D., Ph.D. www.ravnskov.nu/uffe.htm
40. The Holy Bible, King James Version, The World Publishing Company, Cleveland and New York. 1915. matt., 5:37
41. The Food Guidelines 2005 www.usda.gov
42. The International Network of Cholesterol Skeptics. www.THINCS.com
43. The National Academies Press, Nutrient Requirements of Dairy Cattle, 7th Revised Ed. 2001.
44. The National Academies Press, Nutrient Requirements of Dogs, Revised 1985.

45. The National Academies Press, Nutrient Requirements of Poultry, 9th Revised Ed.,1994.
46. Underwood, Anne and Jerry Adler, Diet and Genes, Newsweek, January 17, 2005.
47. U.S. Department of Agriculture. (USDA) www.usda.gov
48. WebMD www.WebMD.com
49. World Medical Association www.wma.net

* The references included in this list are provided for easy access by way of the internet. My desire is for you to review several of the references to access if my interpretation is correct!

This is but a partial list of the literature searched to identifying their position on:

- Mission statements
- Sources of funds
- Research grants supported
- Disease Prevention
- Disease Cures
- Disease Treatments

The Mission Statements sound good but <u>their actions fail to support the mission statements</u> as reflected by the research grants being funded.

Numerous government agencies, (CDC, NIH, etc.) in conjunction with monies raised through fundraisers and other contributions from Industry Partners, are provided to universities and the many foundations who are <u>searching for the cures</u> of the various forms of chronic diseases.

The research grants funded are for finding new treatments (medications or surgical procedures. There is rarely any mention of nutrition or its possible relationship to cause or cure of the diseases.

Prevention of diseases, as practiced, is more nearly directed at avoidance than prevention.

Searching for cures for the various chronic diseases is exceedingly elusive. There is never a search for the cause, which I believe would be a more fruitful search area, leading to true prevention and possibly cures.

They appear to have no trouble in searching for new drugs, new diagnostic techniques or new surgical procedures. Of course, these all offer great financial opportunities for the HOD — compared to the meager rewards, should their research find nutritional changes could provide prevention or cure of the diseases.

Appendix A

New cholesterol guidelines for converting healthy people into patients

Uffe Ravnskov, MD, PhD

In the May 16 issue (2001) of the Journal of the American Medical Association an expert panel from the National Cholesterol. Education Program has published new guidelines for "the detection, evaluation, and treatment of high blood cholesterol" (**read the paper**). Their writing seems to be an attempt to put most of mankind on cholesterol-lowering diets and drugs. To do that, they have increased the number of risk factors that demands preventive measures, and expanded the limits for the previous ones.

But not only does the panel exaggerate the risk of coronary disease and the relevance of high cholesterol, it also ignores a wealth of contradictory evidence. The panel statements reveal that its members have little clinical experience and lack basic knowledge of the medical literature, or worse, they ignore or misquote all studies that are contrary to their view.

Here come a few examples of the panel's false statements.

As an argument for using cholesterol-lowering drugs the panel claims that twenty percent of patients with coronary heart disease have a new heart attack after ten years. But to reach that number

any minor symptom without clinical significance is included.
Most people survive even a major heart attack, many with few or no symptoms after recovery. What matters is how many die and this is much less than twenty percent.
The panel also recommends cholesterol-lowering drugs to all diabetics above 20, and to people with the metabolic syndrome. If you have at least three of the "risk factors" mentioned below, you are suffering from the metabolic syndrome:

Risk factor

Limits according to the NCEP expert panel

- Abdominal obesity: Waist circumference above 88 cm in women; above 102 in men. (Some male "patients" can develop many risk factors with a waist circumference of only 94 cm)

- High triglycerides: 150 mg/dl or more

- Low HDL: Men less than 40 mg/dl Women less than 50 mg/dl

- High blood pressure: 130/85 or higher

- High fasting blood sugar: 110 mg/dl or higher

Test yourself and your family! I guess that using these limits, most of you "suffer" from the metabolic syndrome. And this new combination of risk factors, says the panel, conveys a similar risk for future heart disease as for people who already have coronary heart disease.
Luckily, it is not true.
It is not true either, that cholesterol has a strong power to predict the risk of a heart attack in men above 65. In the 30 year follow-up of the Framingham population for instance, high cholesterol was not predictive at all after the age of forty-seven, and those whose cholesterol went down had the highest risk of having a heart attack! To cite the Framingham authors: "For each 1 mg/dl drop of cholesterol there was an 11 % increase in coronary and total mortality (**115**)."
It is not true either, that high cholesterol is a strong, independent predictor for other individuals.
In most studies of women and of patients who already have had a heart attack, high cholesterol has little predictive power, if any at all.
In a large study of Canadian men high cholesterol did not predict a heart attack, not even after 12 years, and in Russia, low, not high cholesterol level, is associated with future heart attacks (**read summary of paper**
Most studies have shown that high cholesterol is a very weak risk factor or no risk factor at all for old people; see for instance the paper by Schatz et al., but there are many more. Considering that more than 90% of all cardiovascular deaths occur in

people above 60, this fact should have stopped the cholesterol campaign years ago.
Also interesting is the fact, that in some families with the highest cholesterol levels ever seen in human beings, so-called familial hypercholesterolemia, the individuals do not get a heart attack more often than ordinary people, and they live just as long (**read the paper** and **my comment**).
Taken together such observations strongly suggest that high cholesterol is only a risk marker, a factor that is secondary to the real cause of coronary heart disease. It is just as logical to lower cholesterol to prevent a heart attack, as to lower an elevated body temperature to combat an underlying infection or cancer.
It has also escaped the panel's attention that the effect of the new cholesterol-lowering drugs, the statins, goes beyond a lowering of cholesterol. The question is whether their cholesterol-lowering effect has any importance at all because the statins exert their effect whether cholesterol goes down a little or whether it goes down very much.
No doubt, the statins lower the risk of dying from a heart attack, at least in patients who already have had one, but the size of the effect is unimpressive. In one of the experiments for instance, the CARE trial, the odds of escaping death from a heart attack in five years for a patient with manifest heart disease was 94.3 %, which improved to 95.4 % with statin treatment
For healthy people with high cholesterol the effect is even smaller. The WOSCOPS trial studied that

category of people and here the figures were 98.4 % and 98.8 %, respectively.
In the scientific papers and in the drug advertisements these small effects are translated to relative effect. In the mentioned WOSCOPS trial for instance, it is said that the mortality was lowered by 25 %, because the difference between a mortality of 1.6 % in the control group and 1.2 % in the treatment group is 25 %.
When presented with accurate statistics on the value of statins, almost all my patients have rejected such treatment. To claim that the statins dramatically reduce a persons risk for CHD, as was stated in the press by Claude Lenfant, the director of the National Heart, Lung and Blood Institute, is a misuse of the English language.
The figures above do not take into account possible side effects of the treatment. In most animal experiments the statins, as well as most other cholesterol-lowering drugs, produce cancer (**90**), and they may do it in human beings also.
In one of the statin trials there were 13 cases of breast cancer in the group treated vid pravastatin (Pravachol®), but only one case in the untreated control group, a scaring fact that is never mentioned in the advertisements or the guidelines.
It is also an alarming fact that in one of the largest experiments, the EXCEL trial, total mortality after just one year's treatment with lovastatin (Mevacor®) was significantly higher among those receiving statin treatment. Unfortunately (or happily?) the trial was stopped before further observations could be made.

In human beings the effects of cancer-producing chemicals are not seen before the passage of decades. If the statins produce cancer in human beings, their small positive effect may eventually be transformed to a much larger negative one, because side effects usually appear in much higher percentages than the small positive ones noted in the trials.

Whereas possible serious side effects of the statins are hypothetical, those from the previous cholesterol-lowering drugs, still recommended by the panel, are real. Taking all experiments together, mortality from heart disease after treatment with these drugs was unchanged and total mortality increased, a fact that has given researchers outside the National Cholesterol. Education Program and the American Heart Association much reason for concern.

The panel's dietary recommendations represent the seventh major change since 1961. For instance, the original advice from the American Heart Association to eat as much polyunsaturated fat as possible has been reduced successively to the present "up to ten per cent".

But why this limit? Seven years ago the main author of the new guidelines, Professor Scott Grundy, suggested an upper limit of only seven per cent, because, as he argued, an excess of polyunsaturated fat is toxic to the immune system and stimulates cancer growth in experimental animals and may also provoke gall stones in human beings. These warnings have never reached the public.

Furthermore, the panel ignores that a recent systematic review of all studies concerning the link between dietary fat and heart disease found no evidence that a manipulation of dietary fat has any effect on the development of atherosclerosis or cardiovascular disease (**read summary of the paper** -this paper won the Skrabanek Award 1998). For instance, in a large number of studies, including the incredible number of more than 150,000 individuals, none of them found the predicted pattern of dietary fats in patients with heart disease. No supportive association has been found either between the fat consumption pattern and the degree of atherosclerosis (arteriosclerosis) after death. Most important, the mortality from heart disease and from all causes was unchanged in nine trials with more radical changes of dietary fat than ever suggested by the National Cholesterol Education Program, a result that was confirmed recently in another review (**read the paper** and **my comment**). To suggest that diabetic patients should obtain more than 50 percent of their caloric intake from carbohydrates seems unusually bad advice. Many carbohydrates are quickly transformed into sugar inducing rapid changes in blood sugar and insulin levels and thus stimulating a rapid conversion of blood sugar to depot fat and chronic feelings of hunger. Diabetic patients should eat more fat.

Is it a coincidence that the Americans' decreasing intake of fat during the last decade has been followed by a steady increase of their mean body weight and an epidemic increase of diabetes?

Instead of preventing cardiovascular disease the new guidelines may increase the mortality of other diseases, transform healthy individuals into unhappy hypochondriacs obsessed with the chemical composition of their food and their blood, reduce the income of producers of animal fat, undermine the art of cuisine, destroy the joy of eating, and divert health. care money from the sick and the poor to the rich and the healthy. The only winners are the drug and imitation food industry and the researchers that they support.
Uffe Ravnskov
MD, PhD, independent researcher
Spokesman for THINCS, The International Network of Cholesterol. Skeptics

A short edition of the above was sent to the editor of JAMA. Read his answer.
If you lack the scientific evidence of something written above you will find it in The Cholesterol Myths
Feel free to publish this site anywhere, but don't forget to tell from where it comes
Published June 2, 2001; latest revision Oct 31, 2003

Note: For the benefit of those with Internet access, I have left the "hyperlink" listings for your further information.

Index

Series Preview

Book II

Achieving a More Perfect Health (Fall 2006)

This book deals with the various factors relating to health. One should be diligent in their pursuit of better health if they expect to be successful throughout their life. It includes the factors dealing with supplements, foods, weight management, waste elimination, stress management, exercise, plus many other factors. The where and how of achieving a more perfect health will be helpful for reducing the risks of chronic diseases due to malnutrition, as you go through life.

Book III

The Miracle of Eggs (Jan. 2007)

A book that compares the best food in the world, Eggs, with a number of popular foods. There are no bad foods, though some are much healthier than others. The analysis of the different foods is based upon the USDA report on "The Composition of Foods".

The purpose of the book is to dispel numerous myths about those foods that have been deceptively marketed based upon junk science, and have been compared in their marketing efforts to demonize the healthier foods. The per capita consumption of eggs today is less than sixty percent (60%) of what it was in 1945! The health of humans has been devastated as well in this same timeframe, when considering the increased incidence of chronic diseases within the human population.

For information regarding special discounts for bulk purchases:

Contact information:

Harold Rongey

Phone: (714) 624-3029

E-mail: hrongey@dslextreme.com
(or)
drrongey@whostolemyfood.com

R/B Publishing

E-Mail: rbpublishing@whostolemyfood.com

Web Site:

www.whostolemyfood.com